Praise for Ca

"Very few people take the time to delve into the plight of those less fortunate, but Carol D. Marsh takes us into the lives of the women of Miriam's House—homeless, black, and living with AIDS—and gives them a much-needed voice in a sometimes cruel and harsh world. Marsh also reveals with unflinching honesty her own struggles as a white, middle-class woman living and working in a culture unfamiliar and sometimes even distressing to her. *Nowhere Else I Want to Be* is required reading for anyone who wants to know about a side of Washington, DC, rarely seen by tourists or even natives, and a textbook example of the power of the written word crafted by a wonderful writer and even better person."

—Jesse J. Holland, author of *The Invisibles: The Untold Story of African American Slaves in the White House* and *Black Men Built the Capitol: Discovering African-American History in and Around Washington, DC*

"Marsh's memoir deepens the reader's understanding of the complexities faced by women suffering from homelessness, AIDS, and trauma. Her storytelling is vivid and compelling. One cannot enter into the stories she shares without being changed. I could not put down *Nowhere Else I Want to Be*."

—Killian Noe, founding director, Recovery Café, Seattle, Washington

"Marsh writes with joy and humor about her years coming face-to-face with the gritty, sometimes painful, often joyous realities of those we keep on the margins of our society."

—David Hilfiker, MD, author of *Healing the Wounds: A Physician Looks at His Work, Not All of Us Are Saints: A Doctor's Journey with the Poor*, and *Urban Injustice: How Ghettos Happen*

"Marsh was perhaps the most transformative supervisor I ever had, and in my current work I often try to channel her patience and respect for others. I learned many vital lessons during my time at Miriam's House: Conflict is a normal, expected part of life together. Working with women who have been marginalized means you need to constantly be aware of your own broken places. And the best leaders are ones who build trust rather than demand obedience. Marsh was that kind of leader."

—Meridith Owensby, founder and director of
Lydia's House, Cincinnati, Ohio

"I was thrilled to hear that Marsh would be writing a memoir about Miriam's House. The world deserves to know the story of that place, both painful and beautiful, tragic and life-giving. Marsh does a masterful job of sharing the story with her readers from an honest and vulnerable place, never mincing words or glossing over the complicated emotions and situations she experienced while at the helm of the organization. This kind of transparency is a rare gift. *Nowhere Else I Want to Be* is a must-read for anyone interested in a life dedicated to the service of others. Hopefully it will help others to explore their motivation for serving, ask themselves the toughest questions, and ultimately become more self-aware and compassionate citizens— something that is desperately needed in our modern world."

—Cristina Flagg Cousins, MSW

"A woman who climbed the steps to bring hope to women and children. She wasn't on a mission but rather a journey of life."

—Donna Jackson, former office manager, Miriam's House

"Carol D. Marsh actively and routinely sought constructive criticism from her peers and subordinates; this established an unshakable foundation for trust. It also reaffirmed how badly we need each other as allies and mirrors so we can best see how to facilitate beneficial changes for the greatest number of people."

—Christiana Huff, former resident intern, Miriam's House

Nowhere Else I Want to Be

Nowhere Else I Want to Be

A MEMOIR

Carol D. Marsh

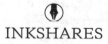

INKSHARES

Published by Inkshares, Inc., San Francisco, California
www.inkshares.com

Edited and designed by Girl Friday Productions
www.girlfridayproductions.com

Cover design by Anna Curtis
Illustration by Emily Davis McCollum
Cover image © DenisTangneyJr/iStockphoto
Cover image © Lava4images

ISBN: 9781942645061
e-ISBN: 9781942645078
Library of Congress Control Number: 2016932413

First edition

Printed in the United States of America

Please Note: Three stories excerpted from *Nowhere Else I Want to Be* have been published in these literary journals: *Soundings Review*, *Jenny*, and *bioStories*.

This book is dedicated to the memory of
all the women of Miriam's House no longer with us,
who taught and inspired me,
and
Robert W. Marsh, my father,
who loved and respected the written word.

CONTENTS

PROLOGUE

I watch the snow come down for hours, rocking and grieving as it covers tree branches and roofs visible from the second-story sunroom. It seems inevitable, falling from a slate sky as though no other weather is possible because I have left Miriam's House. And it soothes me. Under the influence of that blanketed world, grief finally begins loosening its grip. Memories slip in.

Of all the things I could remember about Miriam's House—Claudia's dream, or Gina dancing in the dining room, or Faye nearly being arrested, or Alyssa dying—it's not clear to me why I think first of Kimberly and the mess she embroiled me in a few days before Christmas 1996. But as I relax, it's Kimberly I see. Kimberly watching horror movies. Kimberly insisting she was most certainly not smoking in her room. Kimberly scratching madly at a lottery ticket. Kimberly, drunk, calling my name from outside the house and sounding like a lost soul.

The life I'd participated in and witnessed at Miriam's House had changed me in profound ways. I lived and worked there from 1996 to 2009, fourteen years of life at its richest, teaching me lessons I had yet to assimilate. And so, with memory as catalyst, I get up from my comfortable chair and leave the sunroom for the computer I'd been avoiding for weeks. Perhaps I'm impelled by a desire for catharsis, a need to process my grief and those transformative years by telling myself my stories. It's the desire not to forget, and more important still, not to let the women be forgotten. I begin to make good on a silent wish of some years, and that is to let the world see what I saw: the astounding, courageous humanity of women beset by the worst of societal and physical ills. But for now these thoughts are yet to be formulated. I simply sit down at the keyboard and take dictation from my heart.

CHAPTER ONE

Kimberly pushed through the door I held open for her, stopped a moment to scrawl her name on the sign-in sheet, and started up the stairs when I registered the smell. I rushed behind her, letting the door clang shut on the cold December night.

"Kimberly, I smell alcohol."

"Shut up. Lea' me 'lone."

She was drunk enough to slur even those three syllables. She made it to her room on the second floor before I could stop her, slammed her door, and locked it. I started pounding.

"Go 'way."

Her already deep voice sounded an octave lower.

I told her I'd be back.

"Fuck off."

I ran to my office on the first floor to call Faye, our addictions counselor. We were well into a contentious relationship that would take years to resolve, but I could count implicitly on Faye in situations like this. Miriam's House was primarily a residence for homeless women living with AIDS, but there was a long list of other, equally pressing issues to address, and addictions was at the top of that list. Faye was one of the first staff members I'd hired, a wise black woman in her tenth year of recovery.

We agreed that Kimberly could stay in the house if she gave me a urine screen and promised to remain in her room until Faye could counsel her the next day, Sunday. If not, she would have to leave. Neither of us imagined she would refuse to do what we asked. Since we had opened in February 1996, ten months earlier, we'd had relatively few relapses. The medication then available for AIDS was AZT, which was only minimally effective at holding the illness at bay. Most of our residents were ill enough to make it difficult to get out and score drugs. Of the few who'd managed it, most had, however reluctantly, agreed to give up the screens, stay in their rooms, and then sign a sobriety contract. Those who didn't agree left of their own volition, and immediately.

But this was Kimberly.

I ended the call with Faye, who assured me she would wait for my update. The very thought of tangling with a drunken, profanity-spewing Kimberly scared me. Yet I wanted badly to make her see reason, pee into the cup, and settle down so I wouldn't have to make her leave. I went back up to the second floor.

"Kimberly, it's Carol."

"Go 'way."

Steeling myself, I told her I had the master key and was coming in anyway. Somewhere in the back of my mind was the thought *And just before our first Christmas . . .* , but I put it aside. Still, there surfaced, like a bubble in quicksand, a momentary realization that there was one thing I dreaded more than the drunken confrontation ahead of me: the prospect of kicking her out.

I unlocked Kimberly's door and went in. She was slouching around her room, stormy-faced.

"Kimberly, I can smell it, and you're obviously drunk. But if you give me a urine screen and agree to remain in your room until you can meet with Faye, I can let you stay."

"Don't care."

"You know the rules. You agreed to them when you moved in. You can't stay here drunk unless you cooperate. It's not fair to the others who are trying to stay clean."

"What you doin' up so late? Why you ain't in bed? Go fuck your husband."

"Kimberly, please. If you won't give me a screen, you'll have to leave. It's cold out there. Just give me the screen, stay in your room, and meet with Faye tomorrow."

"No."

"But if you don't, I'll have to make you leave."

I was pleading with her for my own sake as much as for hers, the same reason I was ignoring her profanity. Only the knowledge that I was accountable to other staff and to the policies I had written kept me at it. Left to myself, I surely would have figured out some justification for her to stay.

"My room, can't make me lea."

I had to call Faye again; this was beyond me. As I left, the door slammed shut behind me.

Faye and I chewed over the situation for a long time. We finally agreed that if Kimberly would not leave on her own, I would have to call the police and have her put out. Sick at heart and stomach, I went back to the second floor and took up my position at Kimberly's door.

"Let me in, Kimberly."

She opened the door, scowled at me, and turned her back.

"Kimberly, for God's sake, listen. Just stop a moment and listen. I'll have to call the police to take you out of here if you won't give me a screen or won't leave on your own. Do you understand?"

"Fuck off. Hate this place a'yway. All you mo'fuckers needta lea' me 'lone!" She shouted the last as loudly as her rough voice could manage.

She grabbed a pile of clothing off the floor and tossed it onto the bed, turned and yanked open the drawer of her bedside table. I figured that any more attempts to reason with her would only escalate her rage, so I left to call the police.

I sat on the front stairs, too agitated to do anything else, for the ninety minutes it took the police to arrive. I wanted to be there to let them in, and if Kimberly changed her mind and left, I'd get another chance to persuade her to just pee into a cup and stay in her room for the night. My heart jumped each time I heard the second-floor door open and footsteps come down the stairs, but it was never Kimberly.

When the police officers finally arrived, they were both women, which reassured me. I took them to the second floor. Kimberly was mostly naked when we opened her door to the now routine "Fuck off." She seemed to have been searching for a particular garment, judging from the clothing slung about her room, but why her sodden brain would be focused on sartorial matters at such a time was not at all apparent.

"Is she pregnant?" a cop asked me. It was a side effect of AZT: Kimberly's body was slender, but her belly was distended and bizarre-looking.

"No," was all I could manage, the pitiable sight moving me to tears. This was our beloved, funny Kimberly?

"I hate you, Carol. Di'n't hafta call th' cops. I'da peed for ya."

Speechless, I watched as the officers helped her dress and pack a bag. After they took her out the front door, I went wearily to my office to call Faye and write up the incident report.

"Carol! Carol!"

Kimberly was calling to me, her low, normally growly voice closer to a wail. It was lonely and sad and I had never heard anything like it. The police obviously had not taken her very far, for she had returned to our front door. I'd finished the report, it was late, and I was desperately tired, but it seemed only fair to wait it out. I couldn't leave while she was out there calling my name.

I told myself that Kimberly, streetwise and hardened, would survive. At least, I knew she had survived twenty years on the streets, so I felt assured she knew what to do next. I certainly could not let her in. Kimberly, like all new residents, had heard and agreed to our policies about relapse and its consequences. With the sobriety of the rest of the women to consider, Kimberly's own refusal to cooperate had put her outside our community for the time being.

Yet these thoughts only resonated with hollow and self-righteous justification as I sat immobile, listening.

"Carol. *Carol.*"

Finally, she stopped. I heard nothing more. I left the office, went upstairs to my apartment, got into bed, and did not sleep.

CHAPTER TWO

On February 29, 1996, just ten months before Kimberly flamed out so spectacularly, I had held open our front door as Tamara, the first resident to move in, slowly eased herself up our front walk. With the cold, clear, late-winter day behind her and Miriam's House before her, she stared down at the sidewalk as if it might suddenly shift beneath her. Finally, she had looked up and called, "I'm home!"

A straight-banged, bob-cut wig emphasized her broad face and complemented her brown eyes, looking elegant atop her bulky body that seemed somehow more affected by gravity than the rest of us. As she passed me in the doorway, I noted perfectly arched eyebrows and magenta lipstick.

I remember nothing else about that day, just the way Tamara looked as she came up our walk and the way her greeting rang out warmly. For the rest of that summer and many years beyond, this was how we welcomed women into Miriam's House. We held open the glass-paned front door and in they came, their bags and spirits stuffed to bursting with the detritus of lives lived in defiance of the odds. They came from dope houses, treatment programs, jail, park benches, relatives' couches, hospitals, and basements. They came from lives of abuse and neglect; childhoods lost to poverty, incest, and rape; adult years lost to drugs and alcohol; education lost to low-performing and underfunded schools; self-esteem lost to an uncaring world; trust lost to the deceitful actions of those supposed to protect them; and health lost to asthma, high blood pressure, diabetes, and finally, but not necessarily most tragically, AIDS.

I had first seen the place that was to become Miriam's House in early 1993, while driving around the city looking for abandoned buildings suitable for housing and caring for homeless women with AIDS. I'd already found eighteen possibilities when I first crossed an intersection in Northwest DC and saw the three-story red-brick building on the corner. I pulled to the curb. After so much research, I knew immediately that its long, low profile and relatively small size was perfect. The yard, although just a wide and weedy patch of dirt, allowed for the garden I'd envisioned. The location, near Metro and bus lines and only blocks away from the city's largest AIDS service organization, couldn't have been better. This was Miriam's House.

I found and contacted the owner and got permission for my realtor, development manager, and me to go into the long-abandoned building. As we made a tour, used syringes and years-old trash crunched under our feet. In corners of the apartments lay filthy blankets and rags, discarded McDonald's containers, and other evidence of squatters. Rust and dirt crusted the sinks, tubs, and toilets. It was appalling to think that people had actually lived in this abandoned wreck, but I loved the idea of transforming it from flop house, crack house, and oil joint into Miriam's House. In later years, residents newly sober would point out the basement window through which they'd crawled, back when the building was empty, for a sheltered night's sleep or to get high.

By 1993, HIV/AIDS was the second highest cause of death for black women aged twenty-five to forty-four, and their infection rate was the highest of any one demographic in the country. The virus, called *gay cancer* in 1981 when it first appeared and was as yet unknown, had first manifested itself in homosexual men, so early attention and research focused on that community. But even then, poor black women were becoming its victims in numbers that are surprising now only in that they were ignored.

***

I was in my teens when I had first imagined myself as a benevolent helper of others. I read the book *Christy*, by Catherine Marshall, about a young Southern woman who left home to become a schoolteacher in the Appalachian Mountains, where a woodstove heated the one-room schoolhouse and people lived in shacks with no plumbing. I dreamt of being like Christy and going to work with poor mountain families—later, Indians on reservations, and later still, overseas with the Peace Corps—and helping people who needed me. And there were plenty of people in the world I saw portrayed on TV and in news magazines who were in terrible situations, the cruelty and inequity of which appalled me. I was desperate to make some sense of it all, yet also needed to retreat from it, so I turned to the comfort of dreaming of a life of service in which I would make things perfect for some small village or group of children. For that they would, of course, love and appreciate me. Back then, and well into my life at Miriam's House, my passion for social justice was thoroughly marbled by my need to be liked, causing me much hurt and teaching me things I had no idea I had to learn.

Full awareness of that need and the way it compromised my dedication to justice did not dawn until 1990 when I was in my midthirties and had moved to Washington, DC, to work with homeless pregnant women at a nonprofit called Samaritan Inns. As painful as the growing understanding of my mixed motives had been, those fifteen months at the Inn persuaded me that this was my vocation: living and working with women far less fortunate than me.

In 1996, after three and a half years of wrestling Miriam's House into being, I found myself once more in confrontation with the first of a score of women who would participate in the slow and laborious process of teaching me the meaning of authentic service in the cause of justice.

CHAPTER THREE

To this day, I hardly know how to explain why I founded then lived and worked at Miriam's House. Part of me wishes I didn't have to explain it at all. I wish my choice were as automatically understood as that of a wealthy businesswoman who has risen to a position of power. We understand and relate to the desire for status, wealth, and power, and though we may be jealous or suspicious (Is she selfish? Greedy?) of the rich and powerful one, we live in a world that honors and rewards the accomplishment. So what to make of the one who eschews such things and identifies professionally and personally with the poor and forgotten? Is she a do-gooder? Self-righteous? We wonder, and need her to explain.

But for me, there is no easy answer to the question *Why did you want to?* And in trying to sift through it for myself, I can think of no better explanation for having ended up at Miriam's House than that I was a child of great sensitivity who grew up in the Sixties. This as much as anything else—a middle-class upbringing with my parents' emphasis on discipline, hard work, honesty, and the golden rule—shaped me into the woman who eventually cast her lot with homeless women living with AIDS.

***

When I was seven in 1962, I crouched with my classmates in the hallway outside our room, our heads pressed against the wall and our knees tucked up to our chests. Air-raid drills punctuated my early years with anxiety, making me fearful about what may fall from the sky. At eight I was sent running home from school because President Kennedy had been killed. No one knew if the bombers might be coming, and I sprinted in a panic across lawns and over fences, stomach churning. When I was ten and eleven, it was civil-rights demonstrations, riot police, fire hoses, snarling German shepherds, and murder. It was body bags coming from Vietnam, and stories of napalm burning jungles and villages. I was eleven the year Martin Luther King Jr. and Robert F. Kennedy were assassinated. The story of the My Lai Massacre broke in *Time* magazine when I was fourteen, with its horrific photographs of women, children, and men lying bloody and dead on dirt roads. That same year, the National Guard killed four student protesters at Kent State.

TV images and newspaper headlines of death and violence and war assaulted my heart against my will, horror seeping through as if by osmosis. I seemed to be undefended at a cellular level. This vulnerability fueled what I would later in life call a passion for social justice. And, combined with my sensitivity to the moods, words, and actions of others, it contributed to a rocky start to adulthood.

***

I was a happy kid with a lively curiosity, though shy and introverted. My mother tells me I sang before I could talk, which may have had as much to do with my shyness, inward-turning thoughts, and sensitivity as with love of music and song. As a teen I imagined I was missing a layer of skin, a protective spiritual or emotional dermis necessary in a world that so often wounded me. What protection I did develop came from learning to pretend I didn't hurt.

Yet I was easily hurt, and often by things over which I had no control. My leg would ache when I saw a person on crutches. During a rare family outing to a restaurant, I felt such pity for a man sitting alone and hunched morosely over his meal that I couldn't eat the food ordered for me. Chance remarks by adults and the teasing of siblings could make me cry, which only got me more teasing or an impatient command to stop being such a baby. Exhausted by it all, I craved solitude, wanting nothing more than to find a comfortable nook and read my way out of the world around me: back pressed against the baseboard heaters in the house in which I lived until I was ten; alone in my room after we moved to a bigger house; tucked into the comfortable leather chair in my grandfather's library; or set-tled high in the branches of the willow tree out front. I plunged into books as I plunged into water for the same feeling that later in life would attract me to meditation: weightlessness.

The underwater world was muted, silky cool, and buoy-antly free. It lent me a confidence I felt nowhere else in my life. At nine, I joined the swim team at the outdoor pool behind the office buildings where my father worked. I loved the challenge, even though the competition and intensity often made me so nervous I would vomit, most embarrassingly at the edge of the pool while the children around me scrambled out of range of the splatter. But in the water I had only myself, striving alone.

Rather than lose this feeling, I learned to function at the top of my abilities despite the nausea.

I was the third child of four. My two sisters, three and two years older, were less malleable, more independently minded than me. Thinking the contrast would get me parental favor, I became the helpful one, the good girl, a role that grew naturally out of my cheery disposition and love of peace. Sometimes, though, it made me an insufferable prig, and my quick temper led me to fight bitterly with my sisters. My brother, two years younger, was as anxious to please as I was. We were the wave-smoothers and often allied during any family upheaval.

As the self-appointed Good Little Girl, I made it my job to ensure Mom and Dad were happy. And under the influence of the anxiety I believe I inherited from my father, I was not just good, I was eagerly good, then energetically good, and finally, by about fourteen, anxiously good. I spent my childhood and teenage years learning to be what someone else wanted and needed me to be, so I was often at the mercy of random circumstance or another's whim, habits I would struggle to undo at Miriam's House. Even so, my life was basically a happy one, and I had a creative, joyous energy that brought me to animated engagement with the world around me.

It was as I grew older that I became too absorbed in the happiness of those around me to truly experience my own, or gain much self-understanding. My internal alienation was compounded by a slow-growing belief that I, as the third daughter born instead of the longed-for son, must have been a disappointment to my father. Though I adored him and knew he loved me, I felt the power of his connection with his one boy and knew I was excluded because of my gender. This alone would not have had much power over me had it not been for other experiences making me feel that, because I was a girl, I was unworthy.

When the four kids were introduced as a family, I could see the adults' eyes, particularly the men's, skim over me to settle, pityingly, on my brother. They would say how sorry they felt for him having to live with three older sisters. All the grown-ups would laugh, and my sensitive soul would shrivel.

And then there was the worship and biblical language at the Presbyterian church we attended. There I was told that God loved mankind, had sent his beloved Son to save all men, words of glaring exclusion spoken or read by black-robed and solemn male pastors whose eyes, I imagined, skimmed over me. Once I asked my mother why God loved only men and why was it men, not women, whom Jesus came to save. But her answer—that it really meant all of us, not just men—did not satisfy me because the language didn't change, the adults didn't stop feeling sorry for my brother, and I kept feeling less worthy.

By high school I considered myself a feminist. And I had begun an erratic dance around the meanings of religion, belief, and spirituality, a dance that would waltz me out of and back into church membership for decades. At sixteen I decided I was a deist, after coming across the word in a Taylor Caldwell novel about Cicero. I was a woman-child outside the all-powerful male circles both in my family and in church, and a product of the Sixties' upheaval, violence, and death. Deism made sense to me in a way that belief in a loving and all-powerful God did not. So I embraced the idea that this male god-thing had created the world and then turned away, indifferent, leaving us to our own crazed devices. This early rejection of Christianity foreshadowed years of struggle against and fascination with the tyranny of masculine gods.

As I grew older, the sense of being unworthy by virtue of being female settled in all its unfairness into my psyche. It fueled compassion for all women, and anger at a blind patriarchy whose egocentrism, greed, and lust enabled repressive systems in which women could not flourish while the likes of sex trafficking and poverty could. In this way, my versions of feminism and passion for social justice combined and were ultimately expressed in my work at Miriam's House.

I married immediately after graduating from college with a degree in elementary education. Even though I'd loved college and had done fairly well, I still didn't have the self-confidence to go overseas or even leave my home state of Delaware. Years of searching outside myself for my identity had shaped me in ways that made no room for the courage I would have needed to leave home and family for a faraway teaching job or position in the Peace Corps. The man I married was a single parent raising a small boy, and there I had it: a mission, an unacknowledged substitute for serving elsewhere. What I told myself was love was actually a mutually agreed upon, albeit tacit, arrangement whereby he got a wife, his son got a mother, and I got needed.

I left that marriage after six years, depleted by disloyalty and emotional abuse, and heart-sickeningly guilty for how I had sometimes lost my temper with the little boy, who I then abandoned. I carried that guilt for many years, catching sight of myself in mirrors or windows and watching a smile fade at the unbidden thought, *You don't deserve to be happy.* The choice to leave had been a matter of spiritual and emotional survival, yet I'd been taught that family was of utmost importance, and I couldn't forgive myself for breaking up this one. Leaving the child induced a kind of malevolent self-blame, its toxic effects keeping me from having any meaningful relationship with him as time went on. And that, too, made me feel guilty. It was an ugly, defeating cycle. Eventually, though, it had the benefit of making me more compassionate with and understanding of the mothers at Miriam's House, many of whom had made similar decisions and mistakes.

After the divorce, I studied voice at the undergraduate level for several years, then privately in New York. I still felt more like myself when singing than at any other time. But a cyst on my left vocal cord—from screaming myself hoarse at some long-ago swim meet, I supposed—caused inaccurate pitch in the middle range and made me prone to laryngitis. I quit in early 1990, when I was thirty-five, unsure of who I was or what my calling would be.

I had been attending church in downtown Wilmington, Delaware, with my parents, one of the many times I bounced back to organized religion in my quest to understand life and my place in the world. With the time freed from daily practice and biweekly New York trips, I joined a church committee formed to create an apartment for homeless men. In doing so, I reconnected with the girl who had read *Christy*. I reimagined a life of service, a goal that was encouraged by a new connection with The Church of the Saviour in Washington, DC. I drove south to DC weekly for a springtime course at the church's Servant Leadership School, attended a weeklong retreat in the summer, then took another course in the fall. There I met women and men who had built organizations of varying kinds—for affordable housing, job placement, adult literacy, addiction recovery, child care, and education. These were people to whom I could relate, with a passion for social justice that matched my own and made me feel I belonged.

One of those organizations, Samaritan Inns, needed a resident manager in its Women's Inn for homeless pregnant women. I interviewed for the position on Halloween evening 1990 and moved to Washington, DC, fewer than thirty days later. My family's horrified reaction to the move had something to do with its haste and DC's reputation at the time as the murder capital of the country, but at least as much to do with my own graceless, abrupt, and minimally communicative departure. I'd begun to claw my way free of the good-girl role.

I suffered immediate culture shock, and within a couple of weeks wondered what the hell I was doing there, a suburban-raised white woman ridiculously unprepared for life with city-raised black women. Yet I remained because the work, as difficult as it was, forged a bridge across social and economic divides that so bothered me. In the end, I stayed three months beyond my year, in love with the job and willing to tack on the extra time until they found my replacement.

Eighteen months after that, I was building Miriam's House. To do the work, I crashed through nerves and insecurity, forcing myself to make phone calls, attend meetings, and fight with recalcitrant bureaucrats. These were days when I called upon that skill developed years before at poolside: to function well despite stomach-churning anxiety. Yet much of it was fun and tapped into strengths I'd been developing since those happy years in college: organization, attention to detail, writing, and reveling in learning new things and implementing new plans.

I devoured the only available guide to housing persons with AIDS, published by AIDS Housing of Seattle. I started a Miriam's House newsletter. I learned to write loan and grant applications and then to deal with the group of lenders and grantors cobbled together to fund the purchase and renovation. I formed an advisory committee and began recruiting staff while fighting with the city in the form of one AIDS-fearing bureaucrat who refused even to give me an application, let alone grant a license. I connected with and learned from AIDS clinics and housing organizations. Very slowly, we achieved credibility with city officials, funders, and other nonprofits. Ultimately, Miriam's House became an award-winning and well-respected organization. But that was years in the future, and for the present I had much to learn about myself and about leadership.

And here was the great irony: the leadership skills I had cultivated—taking decisive action and making confident decisions, skills I'd gained fighting inherent shyness and anxiety—were very different from the skills I would need in a community of vulnerable and damaged people, myself included. When Miriam's House finally opened on Leap Year Day 1996 and I stood at the front door watching our first resident approach, I could not anticipate the challenges ahead of me, nor know what Miriam's House and its women would teach me. I would learn to persist in upholding ideals even in the face of my own failure to live up to them, to allow myself to be transformed in the service of a larger purpose, and to find the courage to look first inward for self-understanding instead of outward for acceptance and compliance. I would learn how to maintain equanimity amidst chaos and how to live joyfully into days crowded with life at its fullest. As hard won as those lessons were, the hardest by far undergirded them all: finding within myself the audacity to lead from my own vulnerability.

CHAPTER FOUR

"Miss Carol, it ain't right."

Tamara, just returned from her AA meeting, spoke to me from her position at the security panel in the front hall. In the gray light of the March 1996 afternoon, steadily dripping beads of rainwater plopped softly from the tip of her umbrella onto the carpet. I noted the spreading puddle by her foot, the muddy tracks up the half flight of stairs from the front door, and tried to ignore my mounting anxiety. I was hovering over this building as though it were my firstborn. Besides, this was Tamara, our first resident to move in on our first day a month ago. I so wanted her to like it here. I so wanted her to like me.

But her criticism of our ways in general and me in particular indicated she did not, so I felt tentative around her. And I wondered, *Where was the cheerful woman who'd been so glad to come "home" on February 29?* I liked that woman a lot better. For about a week after she moved in, Tamara had seemed nothing but grateful and helpful. But that had changed as she became comfortable, and she soon displayed an overbearing and sometimes nasty spirit. She would take over house

meetings to berate fellow residents about how trifling (a collo-
quialism I first heard in DC, meaning dirty or unsanitary) they
were, and to needle staff about being too lazy to plan an outing every weekend. She set about—with what seemed to me to
be a gleefully spiteful persistence—disabusing me of my sweet
notions about Miriam's House and how I would live in it. And
though most of the residents were friendly and willing to help
me bridge our differences, I let Tamara's combination of bold
disrespect and sly baiting overshadow all that was going well.

At house meeting: "Why ain't you piped purified water into
the ice maker? Makes no sense to have good water to drink if
we have to put that ice into it. You ain't thinking."

In the dining room after dinner: "You all shoulda heard
Carol in the car on the way to the emergency room when I
had that fever. [Taking on an exaggeratedly sweet voice] 'I hope
you'll be okay. You know I'll stay there with you.'"

But I had to shake off these thoughts because Tamara, in
full cry like a hound after a fox, had not finished with me and
the security system. "I ain't know nothing about this thing,
don't know the code or nothing. What if there's an emergency?"

Her well-manicured finger pointed to the small, LED-lit
panel, part of the system that provided for and monitored the
security of the building: the doors, the sprinkler system, and the
alarm system. Tamara, like everyone else, had an access card
for front-door entry. She could come and go as she pleased,
except for 11:00 p.m. to 5:00 a.m. when the doors were locked
and alarmed. I couldn't understand why she wanted the codes
for turning the alarms off and on. Really, it was a mandated
staff responsibility to ensure safety, not a resident's.

I figured explaining would only bring up more questions,
so I tried reassurance.

"Well, that's why there's staff, Tamara, that's why Tim and
I live here . . ."

She impatiently waved away my words. "Still ain't right. You want me to die in my bed?"

I smoothed the perplexity off my face. What did dying in her bed have to do with it? What did she need from me that I was not giving her? And why was she so changed, so critical?

Throughout the three and a half years of finding, buying, and renovating this building, I'd imagined scenes with the residents: a woman, saved from the brutal street, ill but grateful, telling me about her life while cooking me a pot of greens. Tamara was not conforming to that script.

"Ain't right, me not knowing nothing about this. I gotta feel secure."

Tamara shook her umbrella, scattering drops on the wall and on me. I noticed that her orange nail polish exactly matched the colors in her blouse's geometric pattern. How did she manage that? Wondering if the inner skirmish between my desire to please her and my professional responsibilities was evident in my voice, I tried again. "Well, sure, I want you to feel secure, but we're all trained for emergencies. You'll be safe."

Tamara glared at me from under the bangs into which her rising eyebrows had disappeared.

"Safe?" She spat it out as though I could not possibly know the meaning of the word.

"Give me the code."

Somehow, I managed to untangle myself from that knotty discussion. I left it feeling anxious, frustrated, and upset. Life at Miriam's House was not meeting my expectations.

Tamara was not meeting my expectations.

I was not meeting my expectations. My title was executive director, a role in which I was responsible to the board of directors for everything about Miriam's House: financial health and fundraising; physical plant and maintenance; public relations; staffing and personnel issues; resident care; licensing and inspections; and compliance with a multiplicity of city and federal laws and regulations. I organized my day, ticking off tasks and phone calls in my daily planner, liking nothing more than a list with neat check marks next to each item. These things I managed on my own for the most part, responsibilities over which I had some control, sitting at my desk with the door to my office closed and my introverted self happily busy. And, though somewhat insecure and often riddled with anxiety, I was good at these responsibilities.

All of which was fine for ensuring that Miriam's House, the business, remained viable and even flourished. But there were all these *people* around. With their presence had come a collision between my desire to create a loving and open community and my innate introversion, sensitivity, and defensiveness. That would have been difficult enough had it been all I was facing.

But I didn't feel part of the community I had created, more like a foreigner among these women with whom I had chosen to live. Their vehemence frightened me. Interactions that I thought sounded like arguments were, I had to be told, simple conversations. And simple conversations were often about subject matter beyond my own life experience and narrated in language that made me cringe. I didn't want to judge women whose mode of expressing themselves was different from mine, I really didn't, and had never understood myself as someone who could be petty and biased. Yet my father had instilled in his kids a love of language and a belief that intelligence and culture are reflected in the way we speak and the words we use. My mother, the daughter of British-born parents, was the picture of reticent dignity, keeping strict priorities about morals, behavior, and societal mores. I could not easily shake lessons that echoed in the back of my mind even as I attempted, in the spirit of understanding and inclusiveness, to get beyond them.

And some of my hesitancy was about unkindness: these women could really insult each other. *Girl, them jeans make you look so fat*, or *You act like you from the ghetto*, or *You ain't nothing*. It bothered me to hear women being so cruel to one another, a discomfort that had nothing to do with racial considerations, but with how mean all us women could sometimes be.

I was a peace-loving, steady-the-boat kind of woman living with women whose major communication style seemed to me to be confrontational and often profane, and on subject matter I'd never heard talked about aloud. Safe? Hell, I didn't even feel safe sometimes.

I had never felt so different. So white.

***

I had not known, had not tried to get to know, the only two black students in my high school. Aside from occasionally seeing the black men who took our garbage away, I'd had only one encounter with a black person. It happened when I was just five years old, but the memory is still vivid. I was sitting on a curb in downtown Wilmington waiting for the Thanksgiving Day parade to begin. A black girl about my age sat down next to me. I studied the skin of the little girl's arm— surreptitiously, having been taught it was impolite to stare— admiring its smooth darkness and imagining that, if I touched it, a silky brown powder would come off on my fingers. She seemed beautiful to me, exotic and not a part of my world, yet attractively so. When an adult walked by and kicked up a couple of leaves into my lap, she reached over and brushed them gently away. We smiled shyly at one another.

The 1968 riots after Dr. Martin Luther King's death changed downtown Wilmington and our suburbanite view of it. Shopping trips to Wilmington Dry Goods and attendance at events on Rodney Square ceased. On the few occasions my family did drive into the city, my parents would gravely instruct us kids to close the windows, lock the doors, and keep our heads down so as not to make eye contact. We were not to acknowledge the presence of the newly alien black figures on the sidewalks. I learned to clasp this unaccustomed otherness to myself, hidden and fearful, until a return to the suburbs where I could open the windows, raise my eyes, and breathe.

**

Thirty-five years after a little girl swept a few brittle leaves off my lap, I lived among black women with little clue as to how to connect or how to quell judgments that shocked me even as they popped uncontrollably into my mind. I didn't know how to be genuine, how to stop helping and simply be there. I had never forgotten her, young as I was when we sat on the curb waiting for the parade. And here I was with her sisters out of an urge I could not name or deny, though I believe that child, my first experience of otherness, left such a gentle impression on me as to be at the heart of my move to Washington so many years later. And at the heart of my decision to remain even as I was forced into awareness of a prejudice I never knew I harbored.

CHAPTER FIVE

In quick succession after Tamara, we welcomed Karen and Little Karen, Janelle and Kimberly, as well as two mothers with five children between them. Suddenly, the building that had seemed spacious felt crowded. The community space on the first floor—a well-equipped kitchen that opened to a large and light-filled dining room, which opened to an equally light-filled living room—became the locus of our life together, noisy with its stereo blaring and children racing around, smelling of down-home (meaning fried) food. It echoed with the voices of house meetings, NA groups, AIDS-support groups, and volunteers helping the kids with homework or playing games. Resident rooms, all located on the west end of the building on each of the three floors, began to seem very small and our decision not to build in closets, short-sighted. Our first-floor reception, admin, and nurses offices had a way of overflowing with donations, residents, and the flotsam of community life we had not yet learned to contain.

My husband, Tim, had been excited to move into our apartment on the second floor. I'd met Tim in 1991 after having been drawn to the lay-led Church of the Saviour, attracted by its missions and refreshing lack of dogma. He was volunteering at the church's Servant Leadership School, where we attended noontime prayer, took a class on rethinking approaches to poverty, and were founding members of a centering prayer group. He was tall and slender, with a smoothly long-legged walk, jug ears, blue eyes, red hair, and goatee. Cute. He was also gentle and kind, and as shy as I was leery. It took our friend Sally, in what she freely admitted was a transparent ploy, to get us together. She asked Tim, who had lived in Ethiopia, to introduce us to that country's food. The three of us had dinner at an Adams Morgan Ethiopian restaurant, Sally and Tim keeping the conversation going because it was all I could do, what with my caution and the spiciness of the food, to swallow.

When he later asked if we could walk down to the Mall some evening after class, I said yes. It was not, I told myself, a date. It was just a walk. That was in early summer 1992. We married on July 23, 1993, never having dated, only having walked our way into each other's hearts.

Tim had been raised in the Brethren in Christ Church (an offshoot of the Mennonites), which had a rich tradition of service and generosity to others. His grandparents had sponsored German refugees during World War II, an unpopular move in a community of German immigrants who were trying to stay unnoticed. An aunt and two uncles had given years in overseas missions, and his parents had housed an immigrant from India for a year while Tim was in high school. After college he joined the Mennonite Central Committee, an international relief and development organization. For six years in the eighties, the first three in Bangladesh and then three in Ethiopia, he conducted crop studies and participated in rural development. These experiences in foreign cultures had given him skills that helped him slip easily into place at Miriam's House. And he'd grown up on a dairy farm with its daily chores, seasonal work, and year-round equipment repair, so he was a natural to volunteer for the house's basic upkeep and maintenance tasks, work he relished that connected him with the life of the house.

It all meant that, during those early years at Miriam's House, Tim was better at living in community than I was. For my part, I was happy to have insisted, during the design phase, on an apartment located at the end of a hall and separated by a door and anteroom. That apartment, with its comfortable living space enhanced by bay windows, became my haven, the place into which I retreated with relief when life outside its doors overwhelmed me.

And overwhelm me it did. Often. That first summer was difficult, busy, and confusing. We didn't want to create a cookie-cutter program that forced women to comply or leave, so we opted for an open-to-the-possibilities, organic kind of growth that, while it achieved its goal of allowing the residents to help shape this new program, also left us in chaos much of the time. We found little precedent for what we were doing. Housing for AIDS patients was scarce, and other housing organizations routinely discharged residents as soon as they relapsed, something we refused to do to ill women. When we looked around for a precedent for what we wanted to do at Miriam's House, we discovered we were it.

We began with a few rules about sobriety and violence and being willing to live cooperatively in community. But in short order we learned that, for a group of streetwise and determined and strong women, these three rules, though fine for bottom-line purposes, were far too few. Upon their foundation we gradually built a set of policies and procedures that we learned or had forced upon us by experience and by the women themselves. Women like Tamara, especially. She and

I still didn't get along, and she seemed to want to keep it that way.

Then Janelle moved in to make it worse.

***

I had been enjoying the homey pace of a Saturday morning, a wonderful change from long work days on the phone, at the computer, and in meetings. Sleepy-eyed women emerged from their rooms and headed for the kitchen or the shower. Tamara listened to gospel music while she whipped up her breakfast, making for a joyous noise on the first floor. The personal-care aide (PCA) was busy cleaning the bathrooms, clattering and singing on the second floor. Tim had followed his usual morning routine of hauling trash and cleaning litter from the yard, then bringing in the newspaper and settling in the dining room with a cup of coffee. I was hoping that during the morning I'd have some time to get to know Janelle, our newest resident, who had so far eluded my friendly overtures.

Janelle's eyes, set deep under her brows, were evasive. She had few teeth. Her sparse hair levitated thinly from her scalp. A scowl was her default expression. She seemed to care little about dressing in clothing that matched, let alone covered her. She was negligent with hygiene because she had the beginnings of the dementia that sometimes accompanied later-stage AIDS, although the health-care staff was beginning with some success to foster new habits. Her foul temper, we learned, was aggravated by the toxicity of medications meant to control the onset of blindness caused by a blood infection, but that didn't make it easier to bear. Even the gentlest of suggestions aroused a snarling response, as when we tried to explain to a naked Janelle that it would be better to dress *before* coming to the kitchen for breakfast.

That Saturday morning just after she'd moved in, Janelle needed my help. She had recently undergone surgery for a fistula (a sort of tube of tissue formed between the anus and the skin of her back) and the doctor had prescribed a daily sitz bath. With the PCA busy upstairs, I had volunteered to prepare the bath, hoping it would be an opportunity to connect with her.

I headed downstairs to the storage room, grabbed a small boom box and the prescribed bath salts, scooted upstairs, and slipped quietly into the first-floor tub room just two doors from Janelle's room. I wanted my preparations to be a surprise. Humming, I filled the tub with water at the perfect temperature, emptied the packet of sweet-smelling salts into it, tuned the radio to her favorite station, and placed the bath towel within easy reach of the tub. As I stepped back to admire my work, the door abruptly opened, making me jump to one side to avoid being hit. Janelle came in, grunted at me, and tossed her robe up on the hook. I helped her into the tub and asked if she needed anything else.

"No," she said, not looking at me.

Well, I wasn't going to stand there and watch her bathe. I left, disappointed she'd not acted pleased with the comfy atmosphere. I went to the dining room to check with Tim about replacing a light bulb in a hallway fixture, drank a cup of tea, and listened to the pleasant bustle in the kitchen. After about fifteen minutes, I figured the bath must be over, so I got up to check on Janelle.

The tub-room door opened before I got to it, and out she came. Moving slowly, she gathered the folds of her blue robe about her waist, fumbling with the tie.

"Hey, Janelle!" I called out with bright cheerfulness. "How'd you like the bath?"

She actually snarled.

"I ain't gotta tell you about my bath. I ain't have to talk to you."

With immense dignity despite her unwieldy bulk and the raggedy bathrobe flapping about her knees, she turned away from me and stalked into her bedroom. Before the door slammed shut, she muttered, "I ain't have to make you feel good."

I stood alone in the deserted hallway enveloped in rose-scented wisps of air drifting from the tub room, staring at the door that had closed in my face. Here again, a resident, tough and critical—me, inelastic and wounded. It wasn't her fault, though, that I was so sensitive. Anyway, did it even make sense to be angry with or even hurt by a woman so destitute, so ill? Her personal dignity was about all she had left. I had no right to take it from her or to expect her to behave in ways comfortable to me.

I heard the house stirring around me. I swallowed hard and left for the kitchen.

The kitchen was designed to accommodate a lot of women cooking at once. A ten-burner stove occupied a central island. Perimeter space was large enough to hold a three-door refrigerator, freezer, ice maker, microwave oven, large sink, and dish sterilizer. An open window let in a morning breeze that mingled with the smells of coffee and frying pork. Large as it was, the kitchen seemed crowded that morning. Five or six women dashed about, attending to their pots and skillets.

"Little Karen, your sausage is burning! Better get in here."

"Can I borrow an egg? Thought I had three but only got two. That ain't enough."

"You can have one of mine. I ain't need it right away."

"Thanks. Want some of my grits?"

"Yeah! I love me some grits."

"Miss Carol, what you doing drinking all that tea? You never drink coffee?"

"Nope. Never liked it."

"Shit, who stole my bacon? I know I had a pound in my basket. Ain't there. If I find out who stole my bacon . . ."

"Little Karen, you deaf? I said your sausage burning!"

"Leave her be, Tamara. Here, Karen, I got your sausage. Don't cry."

"Girl, what are you putting all that salt into them grits for? Ain't you got high blood pressure? You about to blow up. Stop that."

"You ain't my doctor."

"If you wasn't so worried about your man liking your food, you'd put that salt away."

"Leave me alone. I can handle my man."

"Them kids should get out of this kitchen with all that running around.

"Right. Guys, it's not safe in here for you, plus you are in the way. Wait in the dining room."

Janelle came in, and my stomach dropped. I moved against the freezer, soothed by the chilly smoothness at my back.

"I woulda give it if someone asked for it. If I find the bitch who stole my bacon."

"Ain't no one want to hear your mouth. Have some of mine."

Janelle stood near the PCA preparing her breakfast. Surreptitiously watching her, I felt some relief that I could detect no upset or anger. Then she came toward me.

"Need my sausage."

She gestured at the freezer door behind me. I moved awkwardly out of her way, struck by her matter-of-fact greeting. After retrieving her package from the freezer, she took it to the PCA and watched it cook. I went into the dining room and sank gloomily into a chair, thinking *Good Lord, I'm just not helping anyone here.*

That thought took me back to my first days at Samaritan Inns, when, in 1990, I had moved to DC to take a volunteer position as resident manager in their place for homeless pregnant women. The shock of moving from suburban Wilmington, Delaware, to inner-city DC had been almost too much for my coddled, sensitive heart. As part of my orientation, I'd been assigned two sessions with Clayton, the addictions counselor. I complained, or rather, whined, about how the women didn't trust or like me.

"I don't get it. I'm just trying to help."

Clayton must have had to deal with many "helpful" women like me. He said what he must have known he was going to have to say as soon as we'd met. "You ain't trying to help. You're trying to get liked."

The memory jolted me bolt upright in my chair, there in the bright sunlight of the Miriam's House dining room. I looked around.

Janelle came in from the kitchen carrying her full plate, noisily scraped a chair out from a table, and sat down. The kitchen door, which I could see from where I sat, opened. Tamara slowly entered and made her heavy way past the stove to the refrigerator. In my peripheral vision I saw Janelle's hand tremble as she raised to her mouth the fork laden with sausage and eggs. I thought about the surgeries, invasive procedures, toxic medications, IV lines, hospital stays, and fevers. I thought about families now distant, women rejected, their fear and shame.

I ain't have to make you feel good.
You're trying to get liked.

CHAPTER SIX

A few weeks later, I sat in the dining room watching Little Karen at the stove. She was a sweet woman, more girl, really, short and slight, gentle, unsophisticated, and childlike. Her face was long and her eyes wide, her smile somewhat tentative. Even her movements were hesitant, as though the idea of thrusting herself into the space around her made her just the slightest bit jittery.

While Little Karen and Tamara discussed what they would cook for dinner that evening, I took a quick look at Tamara, wanting to engage her but still not sure how to do it without incurring her wrath or triggering my neediness. Finally, I just commented on the way her nail polish matched her outfit. She grinned and said she had bottles of nail polish all over her room. They hadn't let her wear it when she was in drug treatment, so she'd bought every color she liked in the early days after she got out.

"Couldn't buy drugs, so I bought polish. That was five years ago."

"You've been sober five years?"

I knew, from the fifteen months I had lived and worked with the women at Samaritan Inns, that sobriety was—no exaggeration—desperately difficult work. I had seen the dogged determination required, the courage to imagine and hold out for a better life when all inclinations were to go back out and use. I genuinely admired Tamara's accomplishment, and told her so.

"Yeah." Tamara regarded her perfectly manicured nails. "When I was drugging, I let myself go all raggedy and trifling. Dirty old sneakers . . ."—she looked at the tattered but comfy Keds on my feet—". . . like yours."

Janelle, seated at the next table, snorted.

"Ripped-up jeans, didn't care about my hair or nothing. In treatment I knew I ain't never want to look like that again."

I ignored the snipe at my shoes and said how pretty she always looked now. She told us how, after the rape (she had been unable to pay her dealer, so he let some guy rape her, and it had been worse than when her cousin raped her when she was twelve) she'd gone crazy in front of a cop and got locked up. The judge had offered her jail or treatment. She chose treatment. Janelle said, "I been raped, too."

"Who ain't?"

Me, I thought.

The morning sun slanted across my lap, warm and comforting. I loved the dining room, so full of light from rows of windows on three walls. It felt simultaneously roomy and embracing. I'd imagined it as a center for family gatherings like those of my childhood. Sunday dinners at home, putting on our best manners and church clothing for the fanciest meal of the week, eaten not in the kitchen, as on the other six days, but in the dining room at the table set with our best silver and china. These meals were what I had missed most when I left home for college, and I'd hoped to recreate them in the dining room at

Miriam's House. Here, like my imaginings about women automatically liking me, was another script that was never followed.

I adjusted my chair to catch the shifting sunlight. Tamara, Janelle, and Little Karen were holding a vigorous discussion about chitlins. I didn't even know what chitlins were. I felt suddenly tired.

Their voices called me from my thoughts.

"I don't let nobody but me clean my chitlins. Ain't no one do it like I do, like my grandma taught me. She was country! She *knew* how to clean her some chitlins."

They laughed. I got up and left.

***

One evening later that week, I was abruptly stopped on my way down the stairs by a peculiar odor. I usually tried hard not to impugn or even give the impression of impugning another culture, but I had no idea that what I was smelling could possibly be food. Mystified, I followed my nose into the kitchen, where the nauseating smell seemed to be emanating from a pot on the stove. I lifted the lid, took a whiff of the steam rising from the boiling mess, and gagged.

Tamara, watching me, grinned. "Chitlins. My favorite."

Oh. It *was* food. And this was Tamara, ever ready with the quick and slicing jibe. I rearranged the expression on my face. "Hmm. Chitlins. What are they?"

"Insides of pigs. Don't worry, I cleaned 'em good. I ain't trifling." She gave the pot a stir, sending another plume of noxious steam into the humid kitchen.

Insides? I wanted to gag again. Watching me, Tamara's smile broadened.

"What you have for dinner?"

"Tofu stir fry." Here was *my* chance to freak out Tamara with an unusual food.

"Tofu? What the hell is that?"

Now I was the one grinning. "Sorta like fermented soybeans."

"And you think chitlins are bad? Fermented beans? Sounds disgusting."

"Not as disgusting as chitlins."

I was a bit shocked at myself for answering in kind. This was not how I usually spoke to the residents. I stole a wary glance at Tamara to gauge her reaction: still grinning. Whew.

"No way my chitlins is worse than them beans." Once she had settled the lid back onto the pot, *thank God*, Tamara turned to send the spoon clattering into the sink, then pivoted back to me. "No way."

"You don't know that. Have you ever tasted tofu?"

She answered too quickly.

"Okay, I'll eat a tofu if you eat a chitlin."

I didn't like where this was going. But her knowing smile galvanized my pride—it surely could not have been my stomach—into agreeing.

Tamara happily went to the cabinet for a plate as I left, rather less happily, for my apartment to get "a tofu." She'd proposed the deal almost instantly, and as I regarded the bit of tofu I'd put it on a small plate, I realized I'd been fooling myself about having the upper hand. At worst, tofu is tasteless, but since my husband had stir-fried it with soy sauce and a few spices, this had a pleasing flavor I couldn't imagine chitlins having. I'd been had.

The tofu and I went downstairs to our fate.

As soon as I entered the kitchen, Tamara grabbed the tofu off the plate, popped it into her mouth, and chewed enthusiastically. Watching me. I stared at her, suspicious.

"At the treatment center they only cooked vegan food. Never did get to like it, but I can eat it."

She swallowed, turned to the stove, and lifted the lid off the pot.

"Okay, and now for the chitlin."

Dipping into the pot, she pulled out a pale, half-curled strip of . . . something. The now-familiar odor sidled toward me. She put the thing on the plate and carried it over to me. I put it into my mouth and my teeth closed on it. Already anticipating the taste, as judged from that smell, I had firmly resolved not to allow my expression to reveal any disgust or, what was more likely, fear. But I had neglected to prepare for the texture, that of a slimy rubber band. Firm resolve, conquered by a chitlin, faltered and fled.

"Acccchhhh!" I spat the offensive thing out onto the plate. "It's like rubber!"

Brown eyes looked at me slyly from beneath bangs. "You have to eat it. I ate the tofu."

She was right. Very quickly, so as not to give my mind or stomach or taste buds a chance to protest, I threw the chitlin into my mouth, gave a couple of ineffectual chews, and swallowed it determinedly—*gagged it down* was how I described it to Tim, later that evening.

Then we went into the dining room, Tamara and I, and we sat down in front of the stereo so she could play her Yolanda Adams gospel CD. The sun was setting, the room in dusk, but we turned on no light. Just the two of us, smelling of chitlins and finding the beat.

***

That June, Kimberly moved in, adding to the mix her signature gruff charm that easily erupted into abusive anger. She reminded me of an elf, or a gnome, maybe, with her short stature and the gamine features that were just as likely—and unpredictably—to be engulfed by a smile as by a frown. She had a pattern of relapsing into drinking, most spectacularly that December evening just before Christmas, with me calling the police and having her put out. And by then she'd already relapsed once before, in the summer, and we'd placed her in the first of several treatment programs.

By July, we had ten residents, three of whom were children—eight, six, and a one-year-old—whose mother was both ill and, in August, relapsing on alcohol and crack. Tamara's heart condition became worse, and she required more procedures and longer hospital stays. Even so, she somehow found the energy for both lovely generosity toward the other women and toxic complaints about staff. Little Karen complained of terrible pain in her head and became lethargic. She was sometimes incoherent, in addition to growing increasingly confused and refusing her medications, although we could not tell if this was due to an unspoken resolution to die, or to her dementia.

A cloud descended on our community. Even as Kimberly and the mother were relapsing and creating havoc, Tamara and Little Karen became sicker. The women who were trying to stay sober were upset about the relapses. And everyone watched, in fear both for themselves and for their friends, as Tamara and Little Karen visibly deteriorated physically and mentally. I became exhausted with the strain of dealing with all the emotions, my own and staff's and residents'. I felt it my responsibility to support and nurture each person, make sure Little Karen and Tamara had regular visits during their many stints in the hospital, and keep the community on an even keel, all the while ensuring the business ran smoothly.

I was overwhelmed. My administrative role had become nerve-wracking in the extreme that summer due to shortage of money. The administrators of the city's funding program—for which Miriam's House had been encouraged to apply and that was essential both for day-to-day operations and for obtaining a mortgage loan—had decided not to open a new round of applications. We would have to wait six months to a year to get operations funding. The Methodist retirement fund, set to give us a mortgage, backed out when I told them. My program director, who had told me when I hired her she was waiting for a job offer from another nonprofit, got the offer she wanted and resigned. Most nights I awakened in a cold sweat with fingernails digging into my palms, fearful of being unable to meet payroll or pay the bills or keep Miriam's House afloat.

Amidst the chaos and difficulties we did find ways to have fun together. Most Saturday mornings the kids and I made pancakes, piling them high on serving platters for everyone to share. Tim took the boys to the park for soccer, stopping for ice cream on the way home. Tamara once ordered Chinese food for the entire community, and a few weeks later, invited all of us to a birthday party her family gave her in our dining room. Adults and kids decorated Easter eggs and on Easter morning prepared a breakfast for which the residents made bacon and grits (food items they told me, accurately enough, I did not know how to cook), while I was allowed to contribute scrambled eggs, fruit salad, and coffee cake. On Saturdays we made clay beads for jewelry, or played Sorry!, Candyland, or Jenga, and popped popcorn for movie nights. The women put gospel music on the dining-room stereo most mornings and danced to the oldies many evenings. Faye, a wonderful addictions counselor who became more beloved as time went on, began what turned out to be fifteen years of Sunday staffing from 10:00 a.m. to 10:00 p.m. She'd meet with the residents, monitor community relations, and cook a dinner that became famous among the women and a magnet for former residents.

We began our habit of piling into a car, and later, the house van, to visit residents in the hospital, carrying plates of food and well-wishes from the rest of the women who were too sick themselves to go. And I promoted Michelle, a personal-care aide with impressive skills and a no-nonsense approach to the women, to program manager. She made a seamless transition into her new work, partly because the former program staffer was generous enough to advise her during her first few months. What had felt like a disaster turned out to be a blessing. Michelle and I developed a strong working relationship.

I was glad for these happy, relaxed times, but most of the time I felt awkward with the women, unsure how to relate authentically. I felt strongly and self-consciously the differences between us and my hidden, I hoped, judgments. And I was very aware, after The Lesson of the Bath, as I began to call it, how much my self-esteem relied on whether I felt the residents and staff liked and approved of me. Was I just one more clueless do-gooder?

Not that there was much time to sit around and ponder that question. When I wasn't in meetings or at my computer or on the phone, I scooted somewhat obsessively around the building prompting and encouraging staff, making sure Janelle had a fluffy throw rug on the cold floor of her room, helping with mopping and cleaning, and trying to contribute to the general quality of life by playing with the kids or cooking breakfast or helping arrange celebrations. I worked what we called duty shifts on some evenings and every other weekend. Long hours in emergency rooms with women in precarious health taught me to keep a tote always ready, stocked with a magazine or book, sweater, and change for the snack machine. I never did find quite the right remedy for my nausea at the smells and sounds of an emergency room. Once I sat with a hawking-and-spitting Tamara, closing my eyes against the sight and wishing there were some way to do the same for ears.

Tamara was in the hospital five or six days at a time, once or twice a month. She endured a procedure to draw fluid from around her heart, and later, needed IV medications for a blood infection after surgery on a forehead lesion. Janelle began to lose her eyesight to an opportunistic blood infection that had invaded her brain. She was put on IV medication, supervised in-house by a visiting nurse, to slow the infection's progress. One of the mothers spiked fevers so high that we took her to the emergency room while scrambling to find care for her three children. Another resident had a stroke and required physical therapy, and we worried about how her legs wobbled even with the support of her walker.

Janelle's visiting nurse left the building one evening without taking Janelle off the IV, causing her to panic, run to the kitchen toting IV pole with lines flying behind her, and fumble so with the needle that it detached and spilled blood on the kitchen floor. Residents refused medications we knew they really needed, or the pharmacy delivered late, or the doctor miswrote the prescription. Each resident had multiple appointments with doctors and therapists and counselors that the nurse monitored, tracked, and recorded.

Life at Miriam's House was busy beyond anything I'd expected. I was teetering with precarious balance on the line between my twin roles of community leader and community member. And there were daily reminders that I was living with women whose life experiences had been so different from mine that we may as well have been speaking different languages, so separate were the realities in which we were living. My upbringing had done nothing to prepare me, nor had life in a neighborhood of families that were, outwardly, at least, just like mine: white, middle-class people living in three- and four-bedroom houses with two-car garages. We all cultivated expanses of grassy lawns with carefully pruned shrubbery. Fathers left for work early in the morning while most mothers stayed home to keep house and, in my case, sew clothing for the family and keep the household accounts with meticulous care. We children attended schools in which almost all the other kids lived the same way, and for most of whom a college education was more an assumption than an option.

I had always lived among people who looked, acted, and spoke like me. I'd been safe, had been taught to trust authority figures, be polite at all times, and help people feel comfortable with me. I loved peace and had never witnessed a real fight, much less participated in one. Almost everything in my life had encouraged me to believe what people said, to trust in their good faith, and to walk out into the world knowing I had a place in it. I was just beginning to learn how differently the women of Miriam's House had lived and how corrosive were the lessons they had been taught by the world and people around them.

Here, I was the different one. I was finding out how uncomfortable that could be.

CHAPTER SEVEN

"Bitch, you keep your slutty eyes off my man or I'ma tear 'em out your head."

"Who you calling a bitch, bitch? Fuck you *and* your ugly-ass boyfriend."

"Fuck you!"

The voices, which I recognized as belonging to Kimberly and Janelle, brought me to a halt on my way down the stairs to my office. They were going at it in the kitchen. This had been building for a week. At least, staff had been telling me it was building. I hadn't seen it, hadn't want to see it. Conflict and I did not get along.

I planned an escape route.

Angela the office manager, whom we called Angie, saw my expression through the glass-paned front-office wall, came out and headed down to the kitchen toward the shouts. I evacuated to my desk, knowing that Angie, born and raised in DC and wiser by far than I would ever be in such matters, could handle it. When she returned in just a few minutes, serenely, not bleeding, I gaped at her. It had sounded like a knock-down-drag-out fight, yet she acted as though she'd just walked to the corner store and back.

"They just needed to get it out of their systems. Didn't mean it."

Didn't mean it? Not how it sounded to me.

She laughed. "You'll see."

And it was not just about fighting. Fun (to me) conversations in the kitchen would turn into appalling (to me) discussions about sex in the crack house. Dining-room chat would get raucous with memories from the street life, including thievery, beatings, and deprivations like being unable to shower for weeks at a time.

"Girl, I can tell you, I was some funky bitch back then. Didn't give a shit. Just wanted my next hit."

Or maybe: "Damn. If that cop hadn't caught me coming out that store, I'da been able to sell that ring on the next street."

And: "That boy ain't had no right to call me out his mouth like that. Simple motherfucker."

Perhaps: "That was the summer I was sleeping on a bench in that little park up there by Columbia Road. Rats everywhere."

And the worst: "Ain't never going home for Christmas. I ain't wanna see my uncle ever again. If I do, I'll kill the fucker. Raped me when I was ten, and kept on 'til I ran away after ninth grade. Ruined my life."

The twenty-four-year-old eating breakfast with me on Christmas morning was explaining why she refused to spend the holiday with her family. The woman in the circle at house meeting had just answered a question about that day's fight with her brother, proud of having stood up to him for the first time in her life. The petite woman with fashion sensibilities so scrupulous that her very shoelaces matched her ensemble's color code laughed a strange, shuddering laugh about those "funky bitch" days. The gravitational attraction between reality and their language held me in the moment. It anchored me in truth in a way my own more elegant and socially acceptable ways of speaking never could.

Miriam's House was, indeed, a strange, new world.

***

In late August, Tamara fell in her room and couldn't get up. Michelle, the nurse, and I attempted to lift her off the floor and onto the bed, but she was too heavy. I left the room to call for the ambulance, the other two staying behind to monitor and support Tamara. When I returned, she had rallied enough to insist we put a wig on her head and makeup on her face. Michelle and I exchanged a frustrated look as she and the nurse left to get the medication list to send with Tamara.

"Ain't going to the ER looking like this," Tamara insisted in a breathless whisper.

"But there's no time, the ambulance is coming and we need to get ready." I was nervously searching the small, cluttered room for her slippers and listening for what I hoped would be the approaching siren.

"Ain't going nowhere without my wig."

The words were whispered, but her tone was unmistakably determined. Impatiently, I spun around and looked at her for the first time since bustling into the room.

Tamara slouched on the floor in the only position that the combined efforts of the three of us had been able to maneuver her—legs splayed out awkwardly, back half-supported by a bed post, one elbow braced on the floor so that her upper body, at least, was semiupright. Sunlight from the window glinted off the top of her head where the hair was nothing but patches of fuzz. She lifted her head, met my eye with an unwavering gaze, and pointing a trembling finger at the wig on her dresser.

I cleared my throat and tried to smile at her. "Next thing, you'll be demanding your lipstick."

"Yeah, that too."

She took the wig from me, shook it, and settled it on her head with her free hand. News that the EMTs had arrived interrupted our discussion about which lipstick—the orangey-red or the purpley-red—would go best with her caftan, but the wig was adjusted and the orangey lipstick applied by the time the EMTs came into the room with their stretcher, medical bags, and masculine, purposeful energy.

Tamara was admitted once again to Howard University Hospital. While she was there, Little Karen was admitted to hospice care (provided at Miriam's House by a professional organization), a decision made by her mother at an emotional cost I could not imagine.

"Please stay with my baby when I ain't here. Please call me when she get bad."

So began the first of many such vigils, attending to life while awaiting death. Bathing, administering pain medications, shifting limbs to ease sore and stiff muscles, changing sheets and plumping pillows, sitting at bedside reading aloud or in silence, grieving in anticipation, our lives went on as usual except for the bedside visits to Little Karen and to Tamara in the hospital. When a staff member called me to Little Karen's room in the evening of the last day of August and I heard the groans, unceasing despite doses of pain and agitation medications, I called Little Karen's mother to tell her to come quickly. She arrived in time for an hour of holding her struggling daughter's hand, saying "I love you" and "Go home, baby, to Jesus." When her daughter obeyed her, she wept.

Together we straightened Little Karen's limbs, bathed her face, combed her hair, and kissed her once more. I gave the bereft mother a final hug at the front door then went back to

Little Karen to set up a table with a lit pillar candle and tea lights. I called Michelle. She drove over from Southeast DC, bringing with her the calm demeanor and air of confidence on which I was coming to rely. We sat together by Little Karen, lit tea candles, and stayed in the flickering dark while residents wandered in and out.

The hospice nurse came, confirmed death, and called the mortician, who arrived within a couple of hours, entering our door in dark-suited somberness. We gathered in the front hall-way and watched in silence as Little Karen's body, zippered into a long, blue bag, was carried out and into the waiting hearse. Then we made breakfast together and discovered that what consoled some—*She in a better place now*—angered others—*Shut up with that!* The flaring anger shocked us into momentary tolerance.

When Doug, my friend who was also a board member and an ordained pastor, volunteered on Sunday to go to the hospital to tell Tamara that Little Karen had died, it seemed a good idea, as well as a relief. He'd been a new Innkeeper at Samaritan Inns when I started there in 1990, and had already volunteered many hours at Miriam's House. His youth group had done a couple of projects during renovation, and had helped to get the place ready for the residents. He'd been around a lot on weekends, so I figured Tamara knew him.

I sent Doug to Tamara, too tired to do it myself. He reported back to me after leaving the hospital. All had seemed to go well. But that afternoon, Tamara's mother called me.

"How dare you get that man to tell my sick baby her friend died? She's stuck in that bed, can't move, ready to die herself. Now she believe she gonna die soon. How could you do that to her?"

All I could do was stammer out my inadequate apology.

Later that same afternoon I sat on the hallway floor in front of my office, talking quietly with a few residents, some lounging on the floor, a few on the stairs. I could see out the front door to the walkway and street beyond, a view I often lingered over. I loved the way the glass door with its glass side panels allowed sunlight to flood the space and the way light reflected off the white walls. It always reminded me that Loretta—friend, off-and-on homeless, and living with AIDS—had repeatedly insisted, during the design and renovation process, "Just don't make it dark. Make it light and airy. Don't make it dark and stuffy."

Usually, I'd imagine I could hear her whenever I sat in this odd gathering place in the building she didn't live to see completed. But on that afternoon, neither luminous cheer nor amiable conversation could release me from the image of Tamara weeping in her hospital bed. So when I saw Faye charge up the front walk, through the door, and halfway up the stairs, the thunderous expression on her face more intimidating the closer it came, my heart sank. I had no energy for another conflict.

Faye and I were already at odds, and I was not really sure why, except that I was afraid of her. She was an attractive black woman with a lovely smile and a talent for storytelling that made me look forward to her sharing at staff meetings. She loved the women and was unambiguously loyal to them. But she was outspoken, vehement in a way that frightened me. And I could tell she didn't like me, or didn't respect me. Whichever it was, the effect was that when she voiced her displeasure, it was with such a tone and such a frown that I would feel myself shriveling like a slug in salt water.

And here she was. Mad.

"Who gave permission for that man to tell poor Tamara that Little Karen died? Why would some stranger go tell her, and not one of us?"

Mad at me.

The residents wanted to know what she meant. She explained while I stayed silent, staring at the floor.

"All alone in that bed, and sick . . . How'd he even know to go over there?"

I felt a light, cold sweat at the back of my neck. Faye must have been angling for a fight with me. She surely knew I was the one who had sent Doug to the hospital.

"Got stuff to do," I muttered as I got up and slipped cravenly away into my office. I would not give her a fight. The residents were there, and I was too frightened to own up. Nothing was possible except, as she glared at me, to make my mumbling exit. I was peace-loving by nature and loathe to fight about anything, and I had no stomach for conflict with Faye.

Even though I knew Doug well enough to be sure he'd been compassionate with Tamara, I realized that his being a stranger to her had unnerved or frightened her. Never again did I allow anyone but myself or a carefully coached staff member to communicate information about the illness, death, or relapse of one of our residents.

During the next few days, Tamara became increasingly confused and had to be restrained, her hands tied to the bed rails so she would not tear out her IV lines. On my first visit to her after this development, I tried to hide my horror, leaning close and putting my warm hand over her cold, bound one.

"Tamara, it's me. It's Carol."

Her bed was next to a window looking out over the parking lot, Georgia Avenue, and then over the rooftops to the Washington Monument, a view she never seemed to notice.

"Going home today. Or tomorrow."

"What? Who told you that?" I was incredulous—she was so sick. I was afraid—we could not handle this at Miriam's House.

"They ain't have to tell me," she said with a flare of her old spirit. "I can leave whenever I want. Going home."

Perplexed, I left her room, telling her I'd be back soon. She didn't seem to notice, sunk in a passivity that was odd for our always observant Tamara. I walked down the clean-'til-it-squeaked tile floor of the hallway that led to the nurses' station. Once there, I waited a bit, intimidated by the piles of patient charts, the ringing phones and clattering keyboards, the absorbed faces of nurses, and the self-important bustle of the doctors, and by my own feeling that I was way out of my league. I finally got someone's attention by simply beginning to speak to the next person whose path on the other side of the counter happened to bring her close to me.

"I'm visiting Tamara in room 223 South. She says she's going home tomorrow, but we have no medical staff to take care of someone in her condition."

I would have gone on, but the nurse lifted her broad, high-cheeked, and darkly smooth face to me and smiled in such a way as to silence me. "She doesn't mean home here. She means home as in heaven."

Without a word, I turned away and walked slowly back down the hall, pausing for a deep breath before entering the room.

"Tamara, honey, I'm back."

"Going home."

"Yes. Yes." I could find nothing else to say as I patted her hand. Go home she did, two mornings later.

We attended two funerals one Saturday that September: Little Karen's in the morning and Tamara's in the afternoon. The memories are preserved in my mind like old daguerreotypes, sepia-tinted in a chilly, rainy September kind of way.

I'm holding open the front door for the women filing past, and they are dignified in their hats and church outfits.

I'm counting heads and blinking away tears as we help one another into the cars.

We are sitting side by side in the pews, the women and I, and I am healthy but they are ill.

I'm struggling to stay calm but nodding and smiling at women—sickened themselves with the disease that made for these funerals—who express concern for my well-being.

We are standing for the wheeling away of a coffin, not once but twice.

Back at Miriam's House, Faye cooked meat sauce and spaghetti, and I made a salad and brownies. We sat together in the dining room for a meal the women called the repast. We told one another stories about Little Karen and Tamara, how Tamara would dress up for the ER no matter how sick she was, and how Little Karen innocently told on herself the one time she relapsed. Faye told us about her new grandson, born on the very day Little Karen died. "A life," she said, and then again, "a life."

I remembered Tamara—*I'm home!*—coming in our door the first time, and understood that I had also, without realizing it, watched her going out our door the last time, wig adjusted and lipstick applied, lying on a stretcher. I thought of Little Karen's final exit, already cold and zipped into a bag. I looked around the dining room at the women whose first entry into our community I had prepared for since I had dreamed of Appalachian hollows and Indian reservations when I was a girl.

I would be witness to it all, and what kind of witness would I be?

We washed the dishes, the women, Tim, Faye, and I. We wiped down the counters and the tables, hauled the trash, swept and mopped the floors. We told one another to sleep well, tomorrow would be a better day. We left the kitchen, the women to their rooms, Faye to her home, Tim and me to our apartment.

CHAPTER EIGHT

The closets in the women's rooms were far too small.

This was good news, actually. During renovation, we'd assumed our residents would live for a few months—eight, maybe ten—and then die. This was how AIDS progressed for most of its victims when monotherapy drugs like AZT and the protease inhibitors were only unreliably effective, as individuals responded to them very differently. But in early 1997, Medicaid began making the new antiretroviral and combination therapy medications available to our residents. Soon thereafter, several of them began gaining health, weight, energy, and interest in life. With improving quality of life came, among other things, increased need for clothing. Hence, our reassessment of the minimal closets we'd stuck up on the walls when we thought the women would need only some robes and soft gowns. In the space of a few months, a carpenter we'd met during renovation designed and built in new closets with mirrored doors.

But for some of our women, the new therapies came too late or were too toxic for their already overburdened organs to handle. We had a decision to make: would we stay with the hospice model, serving only the dying, or would we become a transitional program, admitting women who would improve in health and eventually move into independent housing?

If we stayed with the hospice model, what would we do if a woman we'd thought was declining began responding to the new medications and gaining health? Would we force her out because we served only the dying? And if we did that, where would she go? When we contemplated going with the transitional model, we found we were asking the same question, only in reverse. If a resident who was admitted when relatively healthy began to decline, would we discharge her to die elsewhere because ours was a program for the well? And if we did that, where would she go?

From the first, we had said that at Miriam's House we would meet each woman *where she was*. Originally, this referred to our rejection of what I called the cookie-cutter program, developed before clients ever appeared and written, as it were, in stone. The programs with which we were familiar demanded compliance on threat of discharge. But we were averse to the idea of automatically discharging women in precarious health. Besides, there were few alternative programs for them in DC. Recently, our favorite treatment facility had closed down, and several AIDS service programs had folded due to funding shortages.

Meeting each woman where she was meant treating her as an individual. The three main strictures around violence, drug and alcohol use, and the demonstrated willingness to live well in community—all essential to the basic safety and stability of the house—applied to everyone equally. Beyond that we chose, in a sense, to develop a specially designed program for each resident. This guiding philosophy, already ingrained by the time we were confronted with the hospice versus transition question, gave us our answer: we would do both. Meeting a woman where she was meant that if she declined, she could choose to stay with us rather than leave because we had no capacity to deal with her dying. If a woman became healthier and more engaged with life, she could choose our transitional program with the goal of self-sufficiency and a move into her own apartment at the appropriate time.

Indeed, this combination of hospice and transition had already begun, de facto. Little Karen and Tamara had declined and died at the same time that a couple other women were well enough to attend day programs and go to appointments with minimal assistance from us. Kimberly had used alcohol and cocaine just a month after admission, galvanizing Faye into formulating and implementing an in-house recovery program. Tamara's penchant for acid comment and brutal honesty had led to our creating the first behavior contract with goals for change. Our organic response to the realities of Miriam's House was giving us our answer.

The only questions left were ones we staff members couldn't answer, but had to leave to the residents: How would the women who were hoping to become healthy and independent react to witnessing other residents' deaths? How would dying residents feel as healthier residents announced rising T-cell counts, accumulating months of sobriety, and success in GED classes?

Then there was the irony that was to confound and challenge us during those early years: improved health and new energy for living often meant a return to dysfunction and addiction. A few of the women relapsed even as we enrolled them in classes and day programs, while we were stressing the importance of living responsibly in community. Unresolved mental and emotional health issues, neglected during acute illness, resurfaced, forcing our clarity about what was acceptable behavior. Our compassion for women struggling with AIDS, addictions, and mental-health issues did not mean we would allow abusive treatment among the women or toward staff. Being sick could serve neither as an excuse for cruelty and ugly behavior, nor as a reason for demanding special treatment.

For me, a further irony lay in my own personality and my need for order in my surroundings and relationships. My knee-jerk response to conflict or chaos was to try to shut it down, or flee. But at Miriam's House, where I was in charge and striving to help create a compassionate community, those strategies were counterproductive. Maybe that was why, when there was something upon which I could legitimately impose my will, I did so with fanatic fervor.

***

I jerked my head up, sniffing at the air in my office like a bloodhound on a fresh trail. Smoke. *Cigarette* smoke. Damn it! I shot from my chair, stood under the heating vent, and pointed my nose ceilingward. I sniffed again.

"Someone's smoking in her room!" I shouted to the PCA as I flew from the office. "I'm going to check!"

The ventilation system in our building recycled the indoor air and mixed it with outdoor air, with the result that air from the vent smelled of activities in other parts of the house. We all knew when someone was frying bacon in the kitchen. And when someone was smoking in her room.

Except for roaches, I hated nothing more than residents smoking in their rooms. We had been trying, during fall 1996, to find a place where the women could smoke indoors without endangering other lungs. At first we'd settled on the back stairwell because it didn't share ventilation with the rest of the building. But even making that short trip seemed to be too much for certain residents. Eventually, we had ruled that all smoking must be outdoors and implemented a system of increasing fines: twenty-five dollars for the first offense, fifty for the second, seventy-five for the third and a meeting with staff to talk about finding another place to live. Very few women would ever pay at the second level, and no one ever would progress to the third. But those policy changes were yet to come. So for the time being it was Catch the Smoker.

Stealth was my watchword. I didn't want anyone to hear me and be forewarned. I did not call it sneaking around, as did some of the women. (Smokers all, by the way.) No, this was strategy.

I opened the door to the residents' first-floor wing. I tiptoed down the hall. At each door, the same routine. Move in close, crane neck, twist torso, place nose in optimal position at narrow crack between door and frame. Sniff.

First floor, seven doors. No smoke. Try upstairs.

I slipped through the door to the second floor, listening for the telltale flushing sound indicating a smoker was destroying evidence. No flushing. To the doors, then, nose at the ready. Kimberly's room. Move in close, crane neck, twist torso, place nose in optimal position at narrow crack between door and frame. Sniff.

Aha!

A pause to savor the moment in advance.

I knocked, Beethoven-style. Rap-rap-rap-RAP.

"Who is it?"

"It's Carol."

"Oh." Sounds of quick, furtive movements came from the other side of the door.

I say I know she's smoking in there.

"Uh-uh."

"Uh-*huh*. Kimberly, have I ever been wrong about you smoking in your room?"

Kimberly, when caught at something with no hope of explaining it away, mustered a sheepish charm that made it impossible for me to stay mad at her. She opened the door oozing that charm. "Damn, Miss Carol, how you know?"

I had to smile. "The bionic nose."

"Miss Carol, you crazy!"

She let me into her room. Barely in the door, I choked and gasped theatrically, grabbing at my throat and accusing her of smoking so much that I could hardly breathe. "Where is it?" But even as I asked, I headed into the half bath between her room and the room next door. There it floated in the toilet, a partially smoked cigarette.

"Miss Carol, I promise I ain't never gonna smoke in my room again."

It's a promise we both knew she wouldn't keep.

***

I was being ridiculous, I knew, perhaps even a tad self-righteous, but this was one of the few problems I could address and solve quickly. Part of me actually enjoyed sniffing out the culprit and surprising her in her room. The ensuing one-way discussion—about there being people nearby, including children and adults with asthma or lung disease for whom her secondhand smoke was dangerous—was strongly reminiscent of my father's lectures, a revealing fact I could not cop to until much later.

The smoking problem was solved. Would that others were so easily resolved. Each day seemed to present either a new and unanticipated difficulty or escalating confrontations around a routine one. One of the children was beat up on the playground on a day that his mother was ill, so I went to the school to meet with the principal. We endured an outbreak of scabies originating at a day program several of our women attended. I was beginning to realize that certain hot-button issues—it's too cold/it's too hot, someone stole my food (or soda or bacon or you name it), the kitchen is a mess again, why do we have to have curfews/urine screens/house meetings?—were to be perennials. And I was still unsure what to do, if anything, about the profanity, off-color topics of conversation, and downright meanness I sometimes heard. Who was I to tell these women how to talk?

Then Kimberly found a boyfriend.

Kimberly in a good mood was funny and sweetly quirky. Kimberly in a bad mood was foulmouthed and violently quirky. We saw no wider smile than Kimberly's, no more thunderous frown than hers. She was a woman of broad humor and explosive temper, fun, high-spirited, contentious, and odd. Odd in physique, what with her long, skinny limbs contrasting ludicrously with the fat cheeks and bloated belly attributable to her AIDS medications. Odd in person, with her natural cheer shockingly shadowed by sudden, absolute rages. Kimberly was one of only two women on whom we ever had to call the police, and that, twice. Her quick temper offered entertainment for those who liked to goad her then watch the rocketing fury.

This study in contrasts, this woman with the elfin-faced smile and gravelly voice, at first defied my efforts to become even peripherally acquainted. She was always restless, bouncing from TV room to dining room to smoking patio to kitchen. When I was on duty I had to be content with the occasional quick chat in the dining room or in passing through the kitchen. Kimberly was the perfect prescription for me because she didn't show affection and cared nothing for my need to be liked. She didn't fight me as had Janelle, nor goad me as had Tamara. She just didn't care. When I spoke to her, she typically made do with a one- or two-word response.

I finally discovered a way to connect with her when, during my weekends on duty, I learned how much Kimberly loved horror movies. She tended to stake out the TV room early on Saturday evening so she could watch her favorites undisturbed. Although I hated horror movies, watching them was the sole activity that kept Kimberly in one place for a while, so I'd watch with her until the gore and groaning drove me from the room.

"It ain't real, Miss Carol," she'd holler after me in her rough voice. "It's a funny part coming up, anyway. They chop the guy's head off."

"Well, I'm a wimp," I'd shout back while retreating into the dining room fast enough so I could hear neither the screams bleeding from the TV nor her all-too-realistic narration.

She was patient with me. "It's over! You can come back now."

Two movies she had on video. One was particularly awful, and the other she watched so often even I began to see humor in it. The first was about a murderous doll with a maniacal grin and a penchant for bloody mayhem. The other featured a humanoid grave artifact inadvertently brought back to life by scientists. The thing, no more than two feet tall, would awaken, find a knife, and begin slashing at the calves of any human within range. While doing so, it emitted a high-pitched, hacking shout.

Kyak kyak kyak kyak kyak!

The little guy, relentlessly focused on his prey, would stab repeatedly in what looked like fast-forward motion, shrieking all the while. He was really quite passionate about ensuring the death of any nearby human, and just too funny, with his rapidly jerking arm, the frantic *kyak*-ing, and the slight body thrumming ferociously.

"He's woke!"

On evenings that I was busy elsewhere when the good part started, Kimberly would pause the tape to come find me. I'd rush back to the TV room with her.

Kyak kyak kyak kyak kyak!

And so we bonded, Kimberly and I, over a tiny hellion with a sharp knife and a single-minded instinct for the kill.

Kimberly met Kyle at the Halloween party to which we had invited the men from Joseph's House. He looked harmless and kind of cute—short, slender, narrow-shouldered, and blond, with a perpetually youthful face. Maybe he was harmless. Maybe it was the Kimberly-Kyle combination that was harmful. When they relapsed and Kimberly's behavior changed for much worse, our staff resented and blamed him, which was probably unfair. But we were overworked at the time. Kimberly had begun to spin out of control at a time when several other residents were also struggling. One of the mothers relapsed, and her children, who were dear to us and an important part of the community, left for the month she stayed in treatment. Another resident exhibited suicidal behaviors and asked to be admitted to the psych ward at Washington Hospital Center. Meanwhile, we were trying to complete the urgent admission of a dying woman.

Kimberly stayed out so much with Kyle that there were no more weekend horror movies, no fidgety Kimberly coursing through the house all evening. But when she was present, she fought with other residents and staff. She complained loudly about policies that kept her "in jail." All of her urine screens and Breathalyzer tests had been negative, so, though we were suspicious she'd relapsed, we had no direct evidence. None, that is, until Kimberly herself told us at a house meeting in early November. Not that she realized she was doing so.

Residents and staff gathered for house meetings in the living room every Wednesday afternoon. Sitting in a circle made by moving couches and chairs around the perimeter, we each shared our week's highs and lows, one at a time. Then staff would talk business, make announcements, and discuss policies and rules. Finally, the residents would express concerns, criticisms, and compliments.

At this particular house meeting, Tim had to announce he'd found an empty beer can in the garbage bin at the bottom of the indoor trash chute. Faye, who usually didn't attend house meeting because she had a full-time job elsewhere, was with us that day to underscore the seriousness of this violation of a major policy, and to try and get the drinker to come forward. She may as well have stayed away for all the energy required to ferret out the culprit.

Tim held the beer can dramatically aloft, explaining where he had found it. Then we waited, suspended in a somewhat edgy silence, while the women looked at the can and then away. Faye had barely drawn breath to launch into a lecture about sobriety and the importance of coming clean when Kimberly's hoarse voice stopped her.

"Aw, dang! I thought that chute thing went outside." She sort of grinned and shook her head ruefully.

A pause.

"Girl! You done ratted yourself out!"

I don't remember which resident said it, but the effect was instantaneous. We exploded with laughter. Kimberly froze in her chair, grin gone. Faye stood up and led her downstairs to the staff lounge for a meeting. By the end of it, Kimberly had agreed to a contract including early curfew for a month and an AA meeting every day for ninety days. Perhaps it helped for a while, but Kimberly was still with Kyle, whose allure was far stronger than that of sobriety and quiet nights in the house. We blamed Kyle, fairly or not, for tipping Kimberly over the edge.

And what an edge it was, on that dreary, rainy night just two days before Christmas 1996. Yet as bad as that was, what had made it worse for me was the memory of another woman, another December, and the first time in my life it had been my responsibility to put someone out into the cold.

***

At Samaritan Inns in 1990 I had begun to learn just how different life could be for people not raised in a middle-class suburban enclave as I had been. By mid-December, two weeks into what was to be a one-year volunteer position, I was wondering what the hell I was doing there, attempting to be an authority figure among nine women, all black and raised on the tough and toughening streets of DC. They had struggled and fought for basic survival; I had been given every necessity and then some. They had learned the art of forceful contention; I had learned conciliation. Their defensiveness came of abuse endured; mine of sensitive pride. Their place in society was nonexistent; mine gave me the luxury of rarely thinking about it. Little of this could I articulate then, yet just the sense of it kept me there. I felt the injustice, the unfairness of it all, so out of justice and fairness I stayed, struggling mightily to uphold the rules in a house full of streetwise women who seemed to look right through me to my inner marshmallow.

CHAPTER NINE

The Women's Inn of Samaritan Inns was a place for homeless pregnant women to have their babies and enter into a more stable life. Based on the twelve-step recovery model, as were all of the Samaritan Inns houses, the program insisted on sobriety at the cost of being kicked out, a policy that shocked me when I first learned of it. Before I understood the terrible cost of addictions and how effective the twelve steps of Alcoholics Anonymous and its related programs (Narcotics Anonymous, Gamblers Anonymous, and the like) were, I wondered how the leaders of the Inns, dedicated and passionate in a way that had already deeply impressed me, could send a pregnant woman out into the city. Fervently, I hoped I would never be put in that position. But I was, and very soon after I'd begun the job.

***

The residents had no house key, and the policy was to refuse entry to a woman who had missed her curfew or stayed out overnight without permission. When Denise failed to return one Friday night, I was instructed by my supervisor not to let her into the house under any circumstance. Nervously, I hoped she'd return on the shift after mine so I would not have to be the one to deal with her. But the doorbell rang early that Saturday morning just after I had eaten breakfast and started my shift. I went to the front door with a sinking feeling that dropped through the soles of my feet when I opened it. There was Denise, a half-defiant, half-pleading expression on her drawn face.

I did not unlock the outer ironwork gate. Through its bars I saw her shivering in a thin coat. Beyond her, the December day, dark and cold, curtained in sleet. I, too, shivered.

"Can I come in?" In her brown eyes, a mosaic of despair and hope.

"No," I said faintly. "I'm not allowed to let you in, Denise."

I gripped the iron bars of the gate and peered at her from between my fists.

"Please, please let me in." Against the backdrop of wet, whitening cityscape, she looked and sounded pathetic. The thin coat couldn't cover her belly. Denise had just spent the freezing night on the street and getting high at seven months pregnant.

All I could do was repeat it. "I'm not allowed to let you in."

"What should I do?"

With relief, I remembered what Deborah had told me. "You can go to Deborah's office on Monday morning. She'll tell you what happens next." Any encouraging words I was formulating, all relief I felt, simply died at the defeated look on her face.

She turned away, grabbed onto the bannister, picked her way carefully down the steps and into the somber day. From behind the bars I watched her choose her direction and disappear.

I closed and locked the door and went to my bedroom to sit in silence for a long time.

***

In December of 1996, when Miriam's House had been open just ten months and I sat on the stairs waiting for the police, it was six years almost to the day after I'd watched Denise make her way down those icy stairs. I pictured myself behind the iron bars that kept me inside and Denise outside like the punch line to some ironic incarceration story. I remembered how I'd felt when I learned that she never went to Deborah. I never saw her again. I never knew if her baby had been born healthy. I never even knew if she was still alive.

So while Kimberly's voice came at me from the front patio and before I finally went upstairs, I thought about sending a woman stumbling out into a cold city. I thought about Denise and Kimberly, their freedom to make choices that might kill them, and my choice to be there when they did. The reality of Miriam's House was turning out to be nothing like my romantic, teenage dreams of serving people who all loved and appreciated me because I always did the right thing. What was this ambiguous world in which sending an ill or pregnant woman out into a chill winter night was, somehow, awfully, the right thing to do? The choice to come to DC was one I had made in a semiconscious haze of honest desire to make a difference for the better. Troubled as it was by my need to be liked and the effects of my sheltered upbringing, this choice was landing me in places I'd never anticipated. Places like a cramped crouch on a stairway, sleepless nights, and a corner of my heart harboring indelible memories of a pregnant woman turning away into a veil of sleet and the sound of a belatedly contrite Kimberly calling my name.

It was shocking, the difference between what I wanted my life in service to be and what it was actually turning out to be. Yet the choice to be there was still stronger than the difficulties I faced. When the real doubts finally did come, they would do so after I'd been at Miriam's House for several years. And when they came, they forced me to examine and reexamine not the women's actions, choices, and ways of being, but my own.

***

The day after Kimberly was led out by the policewomen, Faye found her a shelter to stay in until we got her into a twenty-eight-day treatment program. We contacted her several times a week, making sure she had her medications and advocating with the treatment center's staff to allow her to attend clinic appointments. At the end of January, Kimberly finished the program and was on our doorstep, hoping we'd saved her the same room and worrying about Sasha, a newer resident from whom we had not heard since she had walked out after only two months with us.

We admitted two women during February, Kathleen and Muriel, both of them ill and already enrolled in hospice care. Kathleen's was a gentle soul, but she was sick enough that we never really got to know her. She had cancer of the throat in addition to AIDS, and had just finished a second course of radiation treatment that had charred her skin from lower jaw to halfway down her neck. I came upon her once when she was sitting in the dining room looking at the one-year anniversary party photos. She glanced up at me with a wry smile.

"I look like Abe Lincoln."

And she did, at least in that photo, what with her height, emaciated frame, sunken cheeks, and darkened skin giving the impression of a beard.

If Kathleen looked like Lincoln, Muriel looked like an Old Testament prophetess, striding through the house on long, bony legs, her gaunt face aimed at us in shrewd observation. She was the only person I had ever seen whose eyes actually did show a rim of white surrounding the dark iris. And she was so very thin. Were it not for the intensity of that wild-eyed glare, one would think she was about to disintegrate. From her issued a commanding impression of bone and sinew held together by sheer power of will.

I didn't relate to Muriel, I experienced her. The force that was Muriel came at me like a storm front on the open prairie. Nowhere to hide.

She stood up to share during our first anniversary celebration in February 1997, not yet one week with us but as sure of herself as Moses overlooking the Promised Land. With a voice sounding as though it came from beyond our reality, straight and tall, eyes wide, she rambled through a range of topics that were obviously related to each other and to the occasion only in her own mind. I had no idea of the meaning of her screed. And as I glanced around at the other faces in the crowd of residents, staff, and visitors, I could tell that neither did they. We all sat there with that peculiar expression one assumes when trying to listen politely while simultaneously hiding growing concern and marked desire to be somewhere, anywhere, else. I was not the only one who was blown away by Muriel.

***

"Girl, you got big legs! Where you get them big legs?" Muriel glared at me as though personally offended, as though I had worn the legs that day deliberately to upset her.

That hurt my feelings and piqued my temper. Defensively, I retorted, "Well, they're better than those skinny stilts you walk around on." I stalked from the room.

When I saw her later that day, Muriel wouldn't look at or talk to me. Angela, our office manager, told me she'd cried over the insult I'd tossed back at her.

I felt terrible. "Oh no. I did snap at her. But she was teasing me about the size of my legs." It sounded so lame even as I said it. I felt mean. And petty.

"Carol, she was giving you a compliment. She liked your big legs."

I gaped. "I don't want big legs. Who wants big legs? We're supposed to have skinny model's legs."

"Not us. We want big legs, big hips. That's what our men like."

Suddenly I got it. And again I remembered Samaritan Inns.

***

Samaritan Inns. Where it had been, mystifyingly, an insult to be called a skinny-ass. And that wasn't all.

"Wow, you got you some big legs, Carol."

"You showing off them big legs today, huh?"

Embarrassed, I'd just stay silent. Later, I'd fret. Why did they care so much about my legs? And what did they mean, big? I swam and played volleyball all through high school. These were athletic legs. But I became self-conscious, looking at them in the full-length mirror at the end of the Innkeeper hallway, deciding that my ankles were definitely thicker and my calves less shapely now that I exercised less.

Other differences in beauty standards were just as obscure.

"I'm thinking of perming my hair again," I said to Tanya, the other Innkeeper and the first black woman with whom I had ever had much contact. "It'll be summer soon, and my hair just dies in the humidity."

Tanya drew her face up into a frown. "You don't need a perm. Your hair is perfectly straight."

"Well, yeah. That's why I need a perm. My hair is perfectly straight." I looked at her, at the tight curls on her head. I hesitated.

She took up the slack. "We get perms to straighten our hair."

A month or two later, as we were sitting together in the Innkeeper kitchen, Tanya slipped off a sandal and held up her foot for inspection. "Look at my tan lines," she said, twisting her foot to catch the light from the window. "And I wasn't even outside that long today."

Really? Black women get tan?

"Wow," I said, trying not to appear to be the white-bread ignoramus I was.

I filed this new knowledge away with perms that make hair straight. Much later, thanks to Muriel, I was able to add the *big legs are beautiful* nugget. And I began to listen to us women in a new way as we rigorously observed standards of beauty beyond our power to reach, each of us sure we were serially inadequate, and each of us judging the women around us almost as harshly as we were judging ourselves. In this one way, at least, I found little difference between black and white women. We held ourselves and one another hostage to an ideal of physical perfection impossible to achieve.

***

"Should I apologize to Muriel?" I was feeling guilty about snapping at her. "What could I say? That I don't think her legs are that skinny, I was just teasing?"

"No, leave it. She might not remember." Angela seemed a lot surer than I did, but I took her advice and let it go.

"There will be a time to make it up to her this weekend when I'm on duty," I said to Tim that evening as we sat at dinner in our apartment. He looked at me as though puzzled, and I immediately felt the need to justify myself. I gathered my thoughts.

Our apartment had become the haven I needed it to be, the place I felt more at peace than anywhere else. I loved especially the light pouring in from the windows in the large bay, the deep sills that held my house plants. We had plenty of space for the futon sofa, futon chair, and coffee table we'd bought after marrying in 1993, and we'd picked up a round dining table and four chairs at Goodwill. The full kitchen included a stack washer/dryer. In the second bedroom was our computer, my prayer space with altar, bookshelves, and, eventually, a sewing machine. We rarely heard noise from other parts of the house, and residents and staff were really good about not coming to our door.

But we also learned that living where we worked required creating other boundaries than just the physical ones provided by architectural design. This we discovered one early morning just after getting up, me on the toilet and Tim at the sink, immersed in a discussion about some all-consuming matter of business. Ridiculous. After that, we agreed that we would discuss work for no more than five minutes when in the apartment, and then only if absolutely necessary.

This was in my mind as I thought about what to say to Tim about Muriel. I decided to keep it short.

"Well, I won't say anything about the legs. God knows I won't even look at 'em any more. But I can probably make breakfast or do something else to help."

Tim thought I sounded more worried about it than Muriel was. I was already shaking my head in disagreement as he posited that I might not get along well with everybody. I thought about the previous day when a staff member had accosted me in my office to complain that I had not smiled at her that morning when we passed in the hallway.

"I feel like they're watching me, assessing my mood, how wide I smile, whether I treat everyone the same. It's exhausting."

"Do you really think they're doing that?"

"Well, yeah." I tried not to sound too pitying of my intelligent yet clueless husband. I told him about the complaint. And reminded him about staff meetings and house meetings and the grousing from residents about me favoring staff, and from staff saying I favored residents.

"Oh, I don't take that seriously."

He really meant that. All I could do was marvel.

My chance to make it up to Muriel did come that weekend, on Saturday morning when Muriel, too unsteady to make her own breakfast, came downstairs hungry. Elsie, the PCA on shift, had just helped her bathe and dress and was tidying her room, so I offered to make waffles. Muriel said that sounded good.

I found the small, round waffle iron that, as far as I knew, had never been used. I set it on the counter, a simple appliance with just the electrical cord and a light on the lid. No on/off switch and, because it had been donated, no instructions. I picked it up, stumped by its simplicity. How would I know when the waffle was done? Tentatively, I stuck the plug into a socket. The little top light lit up. Seemed straightforward enough. The waffle is cooked when the light goes out.

"Ain't my waffles ready yet?" Muriel called from her chair in the dining room. Elsie had, by then, finished upstairs and come to sit with Muriel. She turned her broad, apple-cheek face and shot me a look as though to signal *She said it, not me.*

"I'm just trying to get used to this waffle iron—never seen one like this before."

I heard no response, though the impatience radiating from the dining room seemed to acquire a distinctly gloomy cast. But I mixed the batter and continued to feel competent right up until the moment I realized quite a while had passed since I'd applied waffle batter to hot iron, and the little light had not yet turned off. I gave the lid a tentative tug. It budged not. Wisps of steam rose from the edges. Had I added too much batter? Cooked it too long?

I waited a bit, then jiggled the lid harder. Reluctantly it gave way, and there was the waffle, a tad on the brown and crispy side, perhaps, but definitely cooked. I made another one and, balancing the syrup and butter in the crook of my arm and left hand, carried the plate of waffles out to Muriel.

"I'll put some more batter in. Just wanted you to get started." I went back into the kitchen to slop more batter onto the iron. As I returned to the dining room, Muriel's voice rose in bitter complaint.

"These is some hard-ass waffles."

I sat down across the table from her as she glowered at the waffles and struck them with a knife. The knife sort of bounced, making a slight *ping.* "Put some syrup on them, that'll soften them up," I said, ignoring Elsie, still sitting next to Muriel and carefully not looking at me.

I pushed the syrup bottle toward Muriel and popped open the lid. She poured a generous helping, watched the amber fluid spread, thumped the bottle down, and stared at her plate. She smacked the knife down again. "Still some hard-ass waffles." Syrup splattered over the tablecloth.

I stood up, reached over, cut the waffles into pieces, and rolled them around in the syrup until they softened. "There. Now you can eat."

And she did. Muriel ate those waffles and the next one, watching menacingly as I smashed her breakfast into small, syrup-soused bites. She ate every last piece, then left for the TV room leaning on Elsie's arm. One final comment floated back to me on the wings of a satisfied belch.

"Them was some hard-ass waffles."

CHAPTER TEN

I seemed to be waging an inner war between my ideals and my inclinations. I loved the fact of living at Miriam's House, as though the teenager dreaming about living on an Indian reservation had finally found her place. Yet I fought the reality of living there when it intruded on my need for solitude and calm, took more energy than I had ever imagined it would, and pounced all over my long-cherished self-image as a compassionate, unprejudiced woman. I wanted Miriam's House to be an open, loving, and honest community that did not shut down disagreement and conflict, but when controversy arose, I longed to run away. Or stamp it out in self-righteous anger. I hoped for teamwork and cooperation among staff, then tended to squelch both because I also thought that in order for them to have confidence in me I should have all the answers. I wanted my staff to communicate openly with me but could get defensive when they did, partly because of the cultural differences in the ways we communicated emotion. These things I knew at some level but was too often powerless over their hold on me. At such times, my only recourse was to retreat to my apartment, grab the rolling pin, and beat on a pillow in an excess of anger that, though it solved nothing, at least dissipated the roiling energy.

But aside from all that was anger-inducing and nerve-wracking—frustration about relationships gone sour, worries about meeting payroll and paying bills, concerns about resident health and sobriety, uncertainty as to how to balance and manage the sometimes conflicting needs of residents and staff—I was slowly gaining confidence in my ability to run the business of a nonprofit. Writing policies and procedures for programs and administration, making charts that would help ensure good record-keeping, strategic planning and problem-solving at board meetings all were areas in which I was doing well even though they tended to raise my anxiety level. I wanted to lead Miriam's House on the path to becoming what seemed difficult for nonprofits to achieve: a mission-oriented and compassionately run organization that was also business-like and viable as a professional entity. I was finding out why it was so difficult. And I was learning that neither Miriam's House itself nor that I had founded and was now running it could make me the woman I wanted to be. Just having seen it into existence was not enough. So much more was being required of me.

At the same time, there were many things I loved about being at Miriam's House. I loved it that I could sit down with a woman whose life had been so very different from mine yet find common ground. On many evenings I could engage in deep conversation with Elsie, the PCA whose wisdom, hard won after leaving the streets to become clean and sober, was deeply spiritual and centered in a way that I craved to find for myself. And all around me were women fighting their demons and choosing to accept the challenges we offered. These examples of courage and the power of human endeavor challenged me and acted as inspiration to keep trying. I began to feel less an outsider, closer to the women because I was seeing the possibility of connecting without judgment at a place known only in the heart, a place beyond culture and skin color. That they were generous enough to let me in, after all my stumbling and tromping about on their sensitivities, was a gift that put to shame the latent snobbery and judgment marking those early days with them.

Even so, and to my dismay, staff relations were proving far more difficult than I had expected. Many of the staff members simply baffled me.

All of the health-care and program staff were black. Tim, the yearly interns, and I were the only whites, making racial and cultural differences ever present yet rarely openly discussed. It seemed to me that my words, written or spoken, were too easily misinterpreted and that my angry flare-ups, for me quickly done and forgotten, were analyzed and worried over excessively. Frustrated anger built up at what I interpreted as laziness and sloppiness. But I didn't know how to confront work performance problems without making things worse. Incipient judgment and superiority bled through my attempts at fair communication.

A case in point was the question of cleanliness standards and how to bring up that topic to PCAs, who tended to the women and kept the house clean, and who already flummoxed me with our widely different styles.

I had discussed this with Nancy, our nurse at that time, and even with her I had felt self-conscious. Nancy, a young and competent black woman, was a good nurse, respected by the PCAs. But she and I were both green as personnel managers. We did not anticipate the minefield ahead of us, laid by history and augmented by our mutual lack of experience and my temper. We came up with what we thought was a good plan.

She would make up a list of tasks to be done on each PCA shift (three shifts beginning at 7:00 a.m., 3:00 p.m., and 11:00 p.m.), and I would create a chart that they would refer to for shift responsibilities.

I called a meeting with the PCAs to review the first draft of the chart and make changes at their suggestions. Nervousness about bringing it up gave me an abrupt and edgy energy. Injudiciously, I began with my complaint.

"I'm not satisfied with the cleanliness of the house."

I ran on about how, when I had made breakfast for Muriel on Saturday, I noticed things that I felt should be done automatically but weren't, like keeping the drawers neat and scrubbing the greasy residue off the stove and microwaves. And that I had noticed cobwebs forming in corners of the stairwell. "It's not acceptable."

The faces of the five PCAs around the table with me had shut down as though quick-frozen in ice. My nerves jumped but I kept going, explaining that Nancy and I had come up with a chart of responsibilities, or tasks, for each shift. I passed out the chart, telling them I'd be back in about half an hour, during which time they could look over the tasks, reassigning them or making changes as they saw fit.

No response. No sort of acknowledgment that I had spoken at all. I got pissed and was not going to stick around. Telling them I'd be back, I shoved my chair away from the table and pushed through the thicket of silence to the door that I barely restrained myself from slamming on my way out.

What the hell was wrong with them?

I stormed up the stairs to my office in a righteous snit and worried that snit for the full thirty minutes, got it by the throat and shook it like a terrier with a new toy. And so was no less full of furious energy, albeit really tired, by the time I went back down to the staff lounge to find out what they'd done with the chart.

I had the small—very small, but at least sane—thought that I should step away from that door and go outside to cool off. But I was too angry. Just as I knocked, a voice filtered through the door.

"It don't matter what we say, Carol will just do what she want."

Even though I heard them laugh when the same voice said, at the sound of my knock, "Oh Lord, please tell me that ain't Carol," I strode, frowning, into the room. I demanded the charts, met no one's eye, and for the second time left in a thick silence. Only this time I was the one with the iced-over expression.

It felt horrible.

Back upstairs in my office, I faced the fact that I'd made things worse. In some way I didn't yet understand, I had not only made myself look silly and weak, I'd handed over a lot of power to these women. Not that I didn't want them to feel power in their work and in themselves, but I'd given them power over me. I felt exposed, vulnerable. I was not earning their respect. I wasn't earning my own respect, for God's sake.

A couple of days later, I was driving two of the PCAs down-town for a training when one asked me, "Carol, you still upset about that chart and all?" I stared out the windshield, concentrated on my driving, and gathered my thoughts. Inexplicably, I felt the urge to giggle.

"Nah. I should have stepped outside to cool off instead of coming into the room. It's over now." It wasn't, but I didn't like the goading note in her voice, and wanted to choose my own time for the conversation.

The other had a try. "You surely got your shorts in a knot over it."

I could have been angry, or at least confronted this disrespectful treatment, but for the time being I was through with anger. Besides, the giggle was rising irresistibly. That phrase, *shorts in a knot*, was just too much. I let the laughter splash through the car.

They said no more.

Nancy told me later what the PCAs said to her about the chart. "It was already printed out. It felt like you'd already decided and they didn't know why you even brought it up. It felt like just another meeting they didn't want to be at where they wouldn't be listened to."

To my mind, I had created a draft, a quickly put together document that we could change as much as needed because it was saved on my computer. To them, it was a pro forma gesture telling them I had already decided. Not to mention that I'd begun the meeting with a cold commentary on the inadequacies of their job performance.

"You're white, educated, and have a lot of power." David Hilfiker, the mentor with whom I'd been meeting monthly for advice and support, was his usual pragmatic self at our next get-together. "They've been at a disadvantage their entire lives, probably barely made it through high school."

David—physician, author, and passionate advocate for the poor—had come to DC from rural Minnesota to practice medicine at Christ House, a Church of the Saviour mission that served homeless, ill men. He founded Joseph's House, for formerly homeless men living with AIDS, the same year I began working at Samaritan Inns. David had told me not long after we met that he thought I might be the person to fulfill his dream of founding a home for women with AIDS. I mark that moment, on a woodland walk at Dayspring, the Church of the Saviour retreat farm, as the beginning of a relationship that became for me more honest, supportive, and valued than any other except that with Tim.

I nodded agreement. "Got their GEDs as adults, mostly, although one never even got to high school."

"Yes, and lived in a world where the people with wealth and power and status who ignore or mistreat them look like you. You represent that other world. You're *from* that other world."

"But I want the jobs done right. I want the work done well."

I got his point, but I had the residents and other realities of Miriam's House to think about. "I mean, it's not like nothing is getting done, but some things are just left, and the rest could always use improvement. That's how I work, constantly trying to better myself, to be excellent in my job."

Suddenly conscious that I was sounding distastefully self-righteous—probably because I was feeling distastefully self-righteous—I shut up.

David told me I was using my schoolmarm voice. He was one of the few people who could speak to me that way without my dropping into a defensive crouch, partly because he didn't make such statements with acrimony or judgment but in straightforward assessment. He said he supposed I'd been raised in a household in which a strong work ethic was stressed. I remembered my dad's fondness for aphorisms, one of which was "A job worth doing is worth doing well."

"You should really listen to what staff and residents are saying about their experiences."

I retorted that I was not *entirely* ignorant of the differences between us and that I was *trying* to be respectful and I *did* want their input.

"And they saw the chart already printed on paper, felt like they were being played, and decided you didn't really care and were going to keep all your own ideas anyway."

Yeah, that was pretty much what Nancy had told me. A sudden, inexpressible weariness settled over me. The gap between my life and theirs, between my understanding and theirs, yawned before me, a chasm chosen by none of us yet on opposite sides of which we stood, peering from behind ramparts built of bitter experience.

"I do want to understand."

He nodded. "Try listening."

CHAPTER ELEVEN

During the fall of 1997, Muriel, already so thin as to seem one-dimensional, lost weight. She weakened and became quiet in a way that reminded me of Tamara. When we asked her what we could do to make her more comfortable, she replied, in her emphatic way, that she wanted a real hospital bed because that hard-ass bed in her room was too damned uncomfortable and how did we expect her to sleep in it anyway? We called her hospice provider, who ordered the hospital bed and reminded us about on-call procedures and the medication-filled emergency kit they'd given us.

Muriel's death was heartrendingly slow.

Our routines anchored us moment by uncertain moment. Into Muriel's room we rolled the wire-shelved wheeled cart that held diapers, soaps, creams and lotions, disposable bed pads, cleansers, room freshener, and extra sheets and towels. On the wall outside her door I tacked the chart we used to track our visits, ensuring that she was not left alone very long, if at all. Staff members completed forms telling me when and how they wanted to be notified of her death. I checked with each resident and kept notes of how and when they wanted to be told. The forms and these notes and all the hospice instructions we kept in a folder in my office labeled "In the Event of Death."

As Muriel deteriorated, we found comfort in these details and activities. Nothing could halt her dying, but I could keep the chart on her door updated. I could double- and triple-check the "In the Event of Death" folder. Nancy and I met twice weekly with the hospice nurses, PCAs kept her clean and comfortable, interns massaged her hands and feet. On a Sunday when Muriel was unconscious, Faye stood at the foot of her bed—the first of so many times stretching into the future that she would do this—prayed, and sang "May You Find Love."

On Muriel's better days, Nancy and a PCA would help her into her wheelchair and bring her downstairs into the dining room to an enthused welcome.

"Muriel! Where you been, girl? Been missing you! Want some of my bacon?"

"I got this new nail polish. Pretty, ain't it? Let me go get the bottle, I'll do your nails. Then I'll do your hair. You got a comb?"

"Miss Nancy, her skin look ashy. Here some nice lotion, put it on her when you take her back to her room."

"Muriel, you comfortable all slouched down like that? Here, let me help you sit up."

When I would enter Muriel's room in the early morning to check on her before going to my office, I'd often find one of the women tiptoeing out, whispering, "She asleep, look peaceful."

Or one who could not bear to see Muriel in her skeletal state and had never so much as peeked through her door, would stop me in the hall to ask if her dying friend had plenty of gospel CDs, or say "Carol, I bought some of that red punch

Muriel like. If I give you a glass of it, will you bring it to her and tell her it's from me?"

Later, when Muriel began to spend all her time in bed, I would find women in her room, chatting, putting a new CD in the boom box, or just popping in for a quick hello before leaving for an appointment. Some would sit with her for an hour or more, watching television, styling her hair, sharing the latest gossip.

Death at Miriam's House was a community event.

One evening about a week before she died, I stepped into the kitchen to see what was going on. Jan, a resident intern, had offered to sit with Muriel for a while, and I was grateful for the break. The kitchen was alive with the after-meal bustle of women washing their plates and pans, wiping down counters and stoves, putting food away.

Kimberly, who had checked in earlier when I was with Muriel, caught me as soon as I was through the kitchen door, worry creasing her forehead. "She so thin, Miss Carol. She ain't got no meat on them bones. Why y'all staff don't feed her more?"

"She's refusing food, Kimberly. It's awful, I know, but she just doesn't want to eat."

"Can't them other nurses make her eat? Them hospice nurses?"

The others in the kitchen, some of them witnessing a preview of their own death, had frozen in place, caught midswipe with a dishtowel, holding a now-forgotten pot or turning down the burner under half-cooked food. Serious and silent, they listened as I explained that hospice care is about comfort, and Muriel had not wanted any feeding tubes or IV needles or hospital. I described how, when Muriel looked to be in pain, when she moaned or frowned or became restless, we gave her pain medication. When she became agitated we had calming medicine for her. The PCAs kept her clean and massaged her limbs so her muscles wouldn't tighten, they changed her position in the bed to make sure the pressure of sheets and mattress wouldn't cause sores. "And we can always call hospice any time, day or night, for advice and support. She's getting a lot of good care and love."

But some still looked apprehensive, so I added, "No one is forced into hospice care if they don't want it. It's your choice, not ours."

A couple of the women exhaled. Relief drifted through the kitchen like an offshore breeze.

"I ain't want it. I want a ambulance, hospital, one of them breathing machines, everything. I ain't ready to die."

"Nor me," someone said.

"And that's fine," I said. "It's your choice. Just make sure Nancy knows."

"Oh, she know all right.

We laughed at Kimberly's vehemence. The somber mood broke on waves of cheer that curled around us and lifted us, for the moment, above fear's cold depths.

Later, when I returned to Muriel's room, I told Jan about the conversation in the kitchen. "I think I'd run screaming away from seeing someone die of the very same disease I had. Yet they visit, they sit with her. They ask how she's doing. Where does that kind of courage come from?"

"I don't know," Jan said. "Maybe it's that they've been through so much in their lives already. Sometimes I think they're so much stronger because of that."

Jan, a petite, thoughtful woman near my age, looked reflectively at Muriel and mentioned that she might be in pain. She'd been moving a lot and had just started to moan. We left the room to find Elsie, who told us it had been long enough since the previous dose of pain medication for Muriel to have another one. But by the time we got back upstairs with it, Muriel was restless and shiny with perspiration.

"Wow, she's real uncomfortable now," Elsie said, going to the head of the bed and smoothing the hair off Muriel's sweaty forehead. "Can you help me turn her after you put that pill under her tongue, and we can clean her up and rub some lotion on her?"

Although she was not heavy, Muriel was tall, with long, gangly limbs. The work felt awkward, bending over the bed at a forty-five degree angle, trying to lift her as gently as possible and without haste. Feeling a rising nervousness, I had to remind myself to breathe deeply and slowly, to will my hands and stomach to soften. Elsie washed her face and fixed her hair. Jan massaged lotion into the skin on her arms, hands, and shoulders, while I smoothed it onto her legs. The small room, crowded with medical supplies, smelling of lotion and dying breath, seemed a holy space. We three women, bending and swaying and reaching like riverside willows over the form so tenuously moored to life, were freed by Muriel's permission to hold her in that spaciousness of love.

But that was not her dying night. Many long nights later, many bathings and shiftings and massagings and soothings later was the night. I wanted to be with her, I'd promised to be with her, when she died. So I sat by her bed for a week of nights, repeatedly dozing and starting awake, then going to my apartment for a few hours' sleep before beginning my work day.

The night Muriel was to die, I combed her hair, settled her head more comfortably on the pillow, and pulled the sheet smooth. Then I sat in the chair at her shoulder and settled my forehead onto the arm I'd propped on the bed rail, too spent to hold up my head. My other hand clasped hers, lying cool and bony on the clean sheet. Muriel had been very, very quiet for hours. The room held a waiting that had nothing to do with me and everything to do with Muriel. Eyes closed, I listened to her irregular, sighing breath.

There dawned in me an awareness of another presence in the room, tall, next to the bed. Momentarily disoriented, I lifted my head thinking the PCA had come in. She had not.

But I had felt it, scintillating, ineffable, and supremely attentive to and serenely heedful of only Muriel. Aside from what I imagined to be a faintly luminous quality to the light in the room, I saw nothing, no one. Just Muriel, long and slight and quite still in the bed. Yet we were three, there in the waiting place, and Muriel was not to be alone for these last faltering steps of her journey home.

***

I looked at a photo of Muriel the other day, of the terribly thin woman with staring, white-ringed eyes and aggressive stance. Of the women I knew at Miriam's House, she was one of a few who really did look as we imagine a homeless, addicted, mentally ill woman with AIDS would look. She was the one we'd pass on the street, averting our faces so as not to encourage any sort of contact. Someone we'd be afraid of and then forget. Yet of the many women at whose bedside I sat during long nights of fluttering pulse and slowing breath, Muriel is the one, the only one, who I can tell you for sure the angels did not forget.

***

I simply could not attend Muriel's funeral. The week after she died, two of the women in the house had surgery, one for a hip replacement and one for abscesses on her neck. I was up and driving to the hospital at five thirty on two mornings. For each,

I stayed until an intern came to relieve me so I could return to work. By the day of Muriel's funeral, I was exhausted and could face no more emotional and physical strain.

What am I doing here? There ensued a time of questioning and darkness that was to last from that October until spring of 1998. It began with Muriel's dying and marched me down the long months of winter through seemingly endless demands on my time and spirit: covering shifts for PCAs and interns who were sick, visiting residents in the hospital, waiting in the ER with ill women for the minimum seven hours it took for over-worked medical staff to treat them. I tangled with the mothers on how to discipline their children and fired the child-care manager after I found her ensconced comfortably in the front office while her charges ran around outdoors, unmonitored. It culminated, finally and horribly, in the intensive-care unit, standing next to the inert body of one of our own.

We were well into our third year. The novelty of those adrenaline-charged reactions to the unprecedented was wearing off, although we still had plenty of precedent yet to be set. The job exhausted me and took every ounce of my physical, emotional, and spiritual energy. Not that having depleted energy was new. But figuring out how to last for the long haul was.

Aside from going to church and its related activities, I had no other life. I was too tired on weekends when not on duty to do more than take long walks downtown with Tim, meandering around the Mall and the monuments, stopping somewhere for coffee and tea, together in a way we could not be while in the community. I stopped going to parties and events—there were too many people who wanted to talk, church friends who wanted to hear about Miriam's House. We two introverts stayed in our apartment, resting, reading, and cooking meals together, glad to allow life outside our door to go on without us for a while.

Tim, having lived overseas in different cultures for six years, was much better than I was at living at Miriam's House. He went about his work with unassuming calm, simply doing what needed to be done without fanfare. I envied him his easy acceptance by residents and staff. Without the leadership issues that plagued me, he could just be in the background doing his job, helping in the community, never the center of controversy as I was. He could just be liked. My pride in and gratitude for his work comingled with an unsettling jealousy and the sneaking idea that not even he could understand what I was going through. In so many ways, despite the presence of Tim and all the staff, I was on my own.

How would I develop the stamina to stay? Because to stay was what I wanted, despite the sometimes extreme demands on my quiet and peace-loving self, despite painful lessons when I was short on compassion and understanding and long on negativity and judgment. I really could not say what was keeping me there. All I could do, when asked, was mumble something about it being what I wanted to do. It was an unsatisfactory answer, and I knew it, yet I didn't know what else to say. If I tried to talk about how much I loved the women and how difficult their lives had been and how it seemed the right thing to do in this unjust world, I sounded trite and pious, even to my own ears. Besides, the answer was simplistic. It ignored the challenges and problems I made for myself. It disregarded those the women made for themselves because survival methods learned on the street seemed maladaptive and served an adult woman poorly in the world of Miriam's House and recovery. How to explain all that?

Yet underneath all the complication was tucked away a rather simple explanation: I simply could not imagine myself living anywhere or doing anything else.

***

Sasha, who had lived with us the previous year but had relapsed and disappeared, returned at the end of October 1997 after calling from the hospital saying she wanted to come home. Kimberly, who had relapsed again in the summer and was at a three-month treatment facility, visited to say she was doing well in the program and wanted her room back when she returned. I felt heartened that they knew they would be welcomed back, that they were ready to accept responsibility for their health and their lives. But Sasha's return thrust us into a maelstrom of conflicting emotions, concern for her mental and physical health, and sheer puzzlement over what was best for her children.

Sasha had come back to us via Washington Hospital Center, where, we found out, she had spent a good deal of time in the eleven months she was gone from Miriam's House. The social worker who facilitated her readmission sent records that showed she'd been treated for heart problems and pneumonia, and noted that she had exhibited signs of depression.

"Carol, why did God do this to me?"

I had just stuck the key into my office door when Sasha accosted me, coming through the doorway from the residents' wing, bundled into in a camel coat and wearing boots for the rainy, cold weather. Well-groomed as always, she had combed her silky black hair into long curls that framed her round, pretty face.

I looked into large brown eyes empty save for pain. "Do what to you?"

"Give me AIDS."

I was too startled to do anything but babble my protest. "No, no, I don't believe for a second, no, not that God *gave* you AIDS." She looked away and began buttoning her coat.

"Sasha?"

She placed a matching cabled hat on top of her glossy hair. She sighed. "It's a punishment, that's what the preacher says. He says God is punishing sins like drugs and all that."

I couldn't have this conversation out in the hallway. I pushed open the office door, telling her to come in so we could sit down and talk. But saying she didn't want to be late for her meeting, she turned away to go down the half flight of stairs, out the front door, and into the windy morning.

Fury at the pastor Sasha had quoted churned through me. I'd heard similar reports from other women. No wonder so many of our residents, gospel-loving though they were, never went to church. What was it with these men, these sanctimonious and judgmental ministers who, black-robed and solemn-eyed, skimmed their eyes over their congregations and told these women they were unworthy to be included in the circle? How dare they?

But I had no energy to take on at a new level my long-lived abhorrence of exclusion and how it riddled the church. I clung to how much I was coming to love Sasha and all the women of Miriam's House. That would have to be enough for now. That, and despairing anger at the stupid, close-minded unfairness of it all.

***

The next time I saw Sasha, I tried to reengage her in discussion about why I did not at all believe God "gave" her AIDS. But she brushed me off. I had to let it go until several months later when, standing in the ICU next to her swollen, intubated form and laying my warm hand on her cold forehead, I told her with complete disregard for her unconscious state she did not deserve this ugly disease, she was lovable and beautiful, and please wake up so we could try again.

But before that, Sasha and Miriam's House had a lot more to go through together.

***

"I can't really tell if she actually wants the girls here. She says she does, and I believe her. But then she make it really hard for Bonnie to bring them even just for a weekend. How would she act if they lived here with her?"

Michelle and I were in the staff lounge puzzling over Sasha and the plan to reunite her and her four-year-old twin daughters. Michelle, a tall, sturdily built black woman with smooth hair falling to her shoulders, had a calm demeanor and the kind of personal presence that commanded respect. Her understanding of the women had quickly made her indispensable to me.

She noted we'd been preparing for this reunification since our first contact with Sasha and her social worker in early September, but since then she had twice been readmitted to the hospital. And we were unsure how steady her sobriety was. To allow the girls to live with their mother at Miriam's House would mean ignoring ill health and tenuous sobriety. And Sasha was not taking care of herself properly, missing doctor appointments and often refusing to eat. She wasn't doing well at managing her own life. How would she manage her daughters?

Michelle considered. "If we do talk about bringing the girls here, it shouldn't be until after the first of the year. That gives her three months to prove her sobriety."

Michelle and I made good partners. She was solid, deliberate in form and manner where I was nervously thin, mercurial, quick-reacting. She had risen above and out of the addict's life and so could understand the women in a way I never could. I had education and a facility with the written word and so could put her wisdom into policies that she could never have written. Although she would leave within a couple of years, outdone by death's constant presence, the work we did together laid the basis for the next eleven years of Miriam's House's work with the women.

I thought her idea about the three-month proving time a good one, and it would also give us helpful information about how well Sasha cared for the girls during their weekend visits.

She jumped at the plan to wait three months until her daughters moved in. The girls' guardian, their paternal grandmother, Bonnie, seemed not so enthused during a meeting we held with her, Sasha, Nancy, Michelle, and me.

"I have a full-time job," Bonnie said, shifting in her chair so that she was angled away from Sasha. "It's really hard to take care of your daughters, *and* work, *and* figure out child care, *and* take care of them when they get sick. I thought we agreed your daughters would live here with you."

Sasha remained silent. Even though I sympathized with Bonnie, I wondered if Sasha resented Bonnie's forceful repetition of the phrase *your daughters*.

Nancy explained that we needed to make sure Sasha's health was strong before we could, in all conscience, allow the girls to move in. Sasha said something, softly, about the headaches no doctor had been able to treat successfully. She did not look up as Bonnie, frowning, reminded her that the girls were hers. "Children should be with their mother."

"I don't feel so well." Sasha, whose personality outside this meeting could be somewhat overbearing, seemed to have undergone a reversal of some sort, her voice hesitant and low. Bonnie began talking about Sasha's son, living with relatives in Texas.

I interrupted. "We can't bring him in here, Bonnie, because our license only allows children twelve years and under. He's thirteen. I understand he's doing well in Texas, and since it's something Miriam's House can't help with anyway . . ."

I let my voice trail off, silenced by the pain on Sasha's face.

Michelle turned to Bonnie with all the force of her practical nature. "Sasha hasn't been well, and we're not sure she would be able to take care of the girls if they were here. And another thing. We need to know she's strong in her recovery. That takes time."

She turned to Sasha. We had agreed that we hated talking about the residents as if they weren't in the room, something that occurred too often and too easily with family members and professionals around. Michelle said again that, although we would love to have the girls in the house, she wanted to see Sasha with three months clean time first. "It's just not fair to the girls to uproot them from where they are now, move them in and then . . . well, I just want to make sure you're working your program."

"I know. I've been going to meetings and all." She spoke up quickly, but her tone was dispirited.

Behind Sasha, on the wall where I'd put it during our first summer, hung a poster: the black-and-white photo of a young woman, with the words "You can't take care of others if you don't take care of yourself first." How few of us women really understood that, and how complicated that simple statement became when we wrestled with what would be best for the children of our residents.

Wanting to reinforce that it was our decision, not Sasha's, and hoping Bonnie would ease up on her daughter-in-law, we explained our policies about children visiting at Miriam's House, that we had to have backup phone numbers in case we couldn't reach Bonnie, and agreements about visit details signed by all parties.

Sasha and Bonnie agreed. I walked them upstairs after we adjourned the meeting. Slowly, diminished in a way I could not name, Sasha said good-bye to her mother-in-law at the front door and went to her room. I returned to Nancy and Michelle, waiting for me in the staff lounge.

"I know what Bonnie meant, children should be with their mother, but it's just not that easy. I mean, it's a great goal, and we should all be working toward it, but it won't do as a blanket statement. I used to think it did. I wish it did."

I closed my eyes. I had just watched Sasha trudge up the stairs, head down. If I felt confused and weary about her situation, what must she feel like?

"You can't blame Bonnie for being upset. She's their grandmother, already raised her own kids. But she's doing a good job. Those girls are always clean and happy."

I nodded at Nancy. "I know, I know. And I do want them to live here. I love having children here at Miriam's House. They just brighten up the place. But only if the mother is able to actually take responsibility."

We closed the meeting, having just spent two hours wrestling with a problem for which we still had no answer.

A week later, Bonnie brought the two girls to our Halloween party, all dressed up and excited. We have a photo of them looking happily over the back of a chair, their little cheeks smeared with makeup and chocolate, their black curls and round, smiling faces so much like Sasha's. Innocent yet at the center of the difficulties swirling about them, they reminded me how imperfect was our ability to influence for the best the lives of the women and children entrusted to us. It was a burden of responsibility that often on weighed me down. But when Sasha's girls wrapped chubby arms around my neck and pressed sticky cheeks to mine, I felt light enough to float away.

CHAPTER TWELVE

The holiday season of 1997 was our second at Miriam's House. Tim and I had parceled out annual family time by allotting a week or two for summer vacation with his family in Canada, Thanksgiving in Delaware with my family, and December— with its holiday parties and Christmas and New Year celebrations—with our Miriam's House family.

Miriam's House had already begun to develop traditions of its own. Michelle instituted the Trim-the-Tree/Decorate-the-House party, always held after a house meeting in early December. Within a week or two of that, we would hold our annual holiday party, to which we invited board members, staff and resident families, donors, volunteers, and other friends. On Christmas Eve, Elsie and I began an enduring tradition. Calling ourselves the Christmas elves, we placed stockings at the residents' doors and piled packages around the tree, many of which were opened almost as soon as we put them down. I took over evening and weekend duty hours so our interns could return home for the ten-day stretch until New Year's Day. I loved the laid-back atmosphere of that week while I hung out with the women and caught up on administrative tasks neglected during busier times.

But the season required that I set aside my shyness and expend what was for me a large amount of energy. The annual holiday party was particularly intimidating in those early years, with its crowd of guests, many of whom wanted to talk with me, and my overly active sense of responsibility for everything and everyone.

So I received quite happily an offer from Michelle and Angela to take over the planning.

"Oh, great. I'd love that. What are you going to do?" Even having accepted their offer, I couldn't resist forcing a plan. "Maybe some sandwiches? We could make a turkey, have rolls and lettuce and tomato, salads and chips. You know, keep it simple."

Michelle laughed and Angie just stared.

"What?" I asked, perhaps defensively, given the laugh and the look.

"Sandwiches and salad? Are you kidding? That's a terrible idea." Michelle, a woman who spoke her mind, had no qualms about criticizing me, boss or no boss. She and Angie explained. Miriam's House would provide a turkey, Angie would fry up some chicken, and Michelle had a great recipe for vegetable lasagna. The women were already talking about making a big pot of greens, some sweet potatoes, macaroni and cheese, seafood salad, rolls, and deviled eggs.

I knew I looked dubious. "That's a huge amount of food. Do you think we need chicken and turkey and lasagna? And all those other dishes?"

Yes and yes and yes and yes.

My approach to celebrations, before Miriam's House taught me differently, was decidedly minimalist. I guess you could say the Miriam's House approach was decidedly maximalist.

***

"That ain't enough balls and stuff."

"And only one box of tinsel?"

"Ain't you bought none of that shiny garland?"

The residents, anticipating the Trim-the-Tree party, surveyed the bags I'd just dragged in from the car. I stopped, unbelieving. The women and most of the staff had complained the year before, our first Christmas, that the tree was too bare. So this year I'd gone to Ames, the local value store, to purchase what seemed to me more than enough to supplement our donated decorations. Really, it all looked rather tacky to me. I clung to the memory of my family's Christmas trees—fine ornaments handed down through generations, popcorn-and-cranberry garlands, tastefully arranged decorations—and was pretty sure this tree would look nothing but cheap. I had even bought a box of tinsel, which I personally thought untidy-looking scattered on a tree, not to mention how it fell off, got tracked all over the house, and then wound around the vacuum-cleaner roller.

"All this? It's not enough?"

Certainly not.

So I went back out to get more, glad that prices were so low at Ames. Under the beginnings of a niggling shame at my snobbery, I decided to stand back and let the community have at it.

Tim assembled the artificial tree on Tuesday night before the Wednesday decorating party. After winding a couple strings of colored lights on it, he came upstairs to tell me that the women wanted more. "Is that okay?"

I told him I was staying out of it. My way of doing things seemed to ruin the fun, and if they wanted more lights, put up more lights. But the budget allowed for no more decoration

expenditures, so we checked in our own closet. Tim grabbed
a string of lights and returned to the living room. Next day in
house meeting, several of the residents thanked Tim while I
squelched a stirring of envy at how easy it was for him to get
approval.

After house meeting on Wednesday, I brought out the
huge can of flavored popcorn and the five-pound box of candy
donated by my mother, a gift she had made to the community both Christmases so far. I put a pot of mulled cider on
the stove, set out chips and dip, veggies and dip, sodas and ice,
cookies and brownies, then went into the living room to check
out the tree decorating.

The room was in a state of disarray that required some
effort on my part to ignore, but I had suffered enough teasing
after the Fourth of July barbecue during which I'd run around
with the Resolve and a cloth, attacking red juice spills on the
carpet. I focused instead on the women around the tree.

"Put this Santa on the top."

"No. Angels go on top. Ain't we got a angel?"

"Got a bunch of small ones to hang on the branches. The
Santa is for the top."

"We gotta put the tree skirt down. Where is it?"

"Here. It's pretty."

"Girl, move aside, we have to fill that bare spot right . . .
there."

"They put out the food. You should go get a plate."

"You mean, I should go get a plate and you'll eat off it."

"So?"

"Where the tinsel?"

"No, don't put tinsel on yet. Tinsel go last, after the decorations and the garland."

"This look just like the tree my grandmother had in her
place."

"We got everything on it? No more decorations?"

"The boxes is all empty."

"Get the garland."

Finally, satisfied that no more bare spots were to be found, the tree decorators joined the house decorators in the dining room to eat so much candy and popcorn and snacks that no one would want dinner that evening.

At ten o'clock, on the final walk-through before ending my evening duty shift, I passed by the living room where a few of the women sat in the light of the tree. I paused, struck by the uncharacteristic quiet at a time when normally the TV would be blaring and a resident or two would be clattering around the kitchen making nighttime snacks or preparing for the next day.

"Hey, Miss Carol, come sit with us."

I sat on the couch next to Sasha and listened to the low conversation and the silence from which it unfolded.

"I ain't had a sober Christmas since I ain't know when. Didn't know it could be so beautiful."

"Nor remembered my kids' presents or nothing. My mother done all that for me."

"All I remember is trying to hide from my uncle. He was . . . nasty." The women nodded and were quiet for a while.

"I'd be dead by now if not for Miriam's House." Nods again. More silence.

"See the way the lights make the tinsel shine?"

"It so peaceful like this. Wish it could be this way all the time."

"Makes me want to put a little tree in my room. I hate the dark."

"Put on that Yolanda Adams CD, the one with 'Oh, Holy Night.' That's my favorite."

We listened. The tree branches sagged under the baubles' weight. Santa listed on his precarious perch. That garish tinsel, scattered willy-nilly and reflecting the colored lights, trembled in the draft from the ceiling vent above, and all of it so beautiful as to make my heart ache.

***

"Did the girls enjoy Christmas here?"

The question was meant to give me an opening with Sasha when I caught her coming in the front door one afternoon just after Christmas. I had read the logbook note written the night before by Heather, our intern. *Sasha said she's not sure she really wants the girls here at all.*

We stood in the front entryway cloaked gray with winter evening. She was, as usual, perfectly made up and stylishly clothed in a short, wool plaid skirt and fuzzy white sweater, leather boots with a zipper up the side. One would not have known her despair unless she lifted her eyes.

"Sasha, can we talk in my office for a minute?"

Slowly she followed me. In my office she sat down on the edge of the chair I pulled out from the table near my desk, and replied listlessly to my repeated question about the girls' Christmas. She stared at the floor past fingers interlaced on her lap. Her head was so low her face was only partly visible behind a drapery of dark curls.

A slight noise. I looked up. And she said to me, "I feel my life slipping away."

She recited the litany of ills—constant headache, doctors poking and prodding, tired, always tired, heart bad, pneumonia again and again.

"I feel my life slipping away," she repeated.

***

And so later that week, Nancy, Michelle, Sasha, and I met with Bonnie to make arrangements for Bonnie to adopt Sasha's twin daughters. We had thought this would ease Sasha's stress, and we'd hoped to see an improvement in temper, a return to funny, engaged Sasha. Instead, she remained wrapped in something impenetrable to us, as though a grim troll had trapped her inside a malevolent spell.

In February we gave Nancy, who was marrying and moving away, a wedding shower. A few weeks after that, Sasha disappeared. Frantic, we called hospitals, we called Bonnie, we called her case manager, we called her friends. We could not find her. We feared she'd relapsed and was out there using as she had been the year before.

Kathy, the nurse we'd just hired to take Nancy's place, told me that on a recent afternoon she'd been driving Sasha down Fourteenth Street when they'd passed Central Union Mission. Outside the building, in a line curving around the corner and down the street, were the men waiting for their evening meal. Sasha, staring out of the car window, had muttered, "Look at that, all those wasted lives." It was the only thing she said aloud that afternoon.

In early March, Angie called out to me from her desk in the front office that Washington Hospital Center was on the phone about Sasha. She came into my office, looking hopeful, as I picked up the transferred call. The social worker who had placed Sasha at Miriam's House the previous fall told me Sasha had been admitted. Angie rushed away to get interns, and I said we'd have someone there right away. Michelle called Bonnie. We delegated Jan and Heather, the newest resident intern, to go to Sasha. Then for the next half hour Michelle, Angie, and I tried to work but mainly stared at the phone as though willing it to ring, not knowing the call, when it came, would devastate us.

"Carol, we're coming back. It's awful." Jan's voice broke. "She's in the intensive-care unit, on that breathing machine. She's unconscious, didn't even know we were there."

As soon as Heather and Jan returned, I took the car and drove to Washington Hospital Center.

I had never before seen an intubated person. Her body was swollen, her skin cold, face bloated, and cheeks covered with blood-stained tape holding in place the tube stretching her mouth into a tight, uneven grimace. I might not have recognized her had I not been told it was her.

"She had a lot of drugs in her system when we admitted her." I looked up to see the doctor who had entered while I stood beside Sasha lost in pained contemplation, her defensive tone possibly a reaction to the expression on my face. She looked at the chart resting on her forearm. "Her organs have shut down, and we don't know how to reach her family. If you know them, tell them they should get here right away."

She left, still focused on the chart, and I turned back to Sasha, listening to the hiss of the ventilator that kept time with the rise and fall of her chest.

My life is slipping away.

Back at the house a half hour later, the women, warned by Angie and Michelle, were waiting.

"You want to know how she is?" I asked, too grief-stricken to modulate my words. "She's basically dead, she's breathing because a machine is making air go into her lungs, and she doesn't know who we are or even that we're there. That's how she is, and the doctor said her body was full of drugs when she came in."

My voice, I knew, was harsh, choking. Around me in the circle of shocked women were those beloved to me whose next relapse might destroy them. For once I didn't care if they liked what I said or that they might be mad at my speaking so bluntly. "It turns out that there actually *is* one last relapse that will kill you."

Still, they wanted to visit Sasha. Still, they waited while I got something to eat. Still, they patted my arm and murmured when I told them to dress warmly because the afternoon had turned cold, "Don't worry, Miss Carol, it gonna be all right."

Two by two we visited her, the bulk of our group in the waiting room. Kimberly had brought her Bible. She read to Sasha her own favorite, Psalm 23. Two at a time we said good-bye. We patted the cold, swollen hand. We stumbled a bit as we walked away.

Her mother had Sasha cremated. We attended the memorial service, with its large photo of beautiful, laughing Sasha on an easel at the front of the chapel, and her daughters, uncomprehending, dressed in pretty black dresses with lace collars, happy to see us and clamoring to climb into our laps. After the service ended, Bonnie gave us all hugs and told us she was doing well with the twins. We saw her and the girls no more.

CHAPTER THIRTEEN

Spring 1998, the start of our third year, brought the beginning of a period of relative calm. Staff were settling into jobs made meaningful by death and more do-able with accumulated experience. I felt less wary of delegating. Angie was proving to be a valuable resource for understanding the women as well as a good office manager. Jan was in her second year with us, taking on extra responsibilities and lifting a few from my shoulders. A deeply spiritual and empathic woman, she provided much-needed support to me. Heather had a calm dignity that worked well in our often chaotic house. She had a work ethic like my own, only she seemed a lot less anxious about it. With Jan and Heather taking most duty nights and weekends, I had less work to do in the community and more time to rest.

The residents—nine women and a mother with two girls in elementary school—comprised a fairly stable bunch, working their programs, sharing cooking and cleanup, helping with the children, teaching the newer residents about AIDS, and encouraging one another in recovery.

We gave a surprise shower for our new nurse, Kathy, who was to marry in April, much of it planned and prepared by the women. The two little girls and their mother helped me cook Mother's Day breakfast, and later that week most of the community gathered in the TV room to watch the final *Seinfeld* episode. Kimberly dyed her hair a startling blond, then accepted with good nature the teasing that trailed after her for a week or so. A Memorial Day picnic at the house featured one woman grilling the chicken pieces and spare ribs another had prepared. One made deviled eggs; Karen made macaroni and tuna salad; Jan, pork and beans; and me, brownies. Kimberly appeared in time to eat and then vanished before cleanup began, making her the focus of strident complaint about her laziness at the next house meeting.

In June 1998, the development director I had hired two years before left for a mission trip to Yugoslavia. Tim left his job with another nonprofit organization to take the position, something David had recommended to us a year before. I would be his boss, and we thought we could manage the unusual relationship, but agreed with the board that we would take a second look at the decision in six months and report back.

Two of the residents who had some training as hair stylists made the TV room their salon until complaints about the smell and the tracks (which, I learned, were lengths of hair to be glued to the scalp) all over the furniture forced them out. They moved operations to the ground-floor rec room, down the hall from the laundry room's hair-washing sink. We celebrated Tonia's one-year anniversary with cake and dancing. At the party, Kimberly tried to teach Jan how to dance but gave up with the unoriginal comment that white women couldn't dance, a criticism Jan said was only too true, at least in her case. We all went to the circus and then listened in house meeting when two of the women shared that it felt like they were seeing a circus for the first time because they were seeing it sober for the first time. Jan arranged movie outings most Saturdays, Heather brought in a group to conduct health and safer sex workshops, and I developed the habit of cooking Sunday breakfast every week as long as someone else would fry up the bacon.

For Tim and me, this respite from the outsize emotions and complications of the previous ten months was a welcome opportunity to settle more deeply into our life as part of the community. Tim started painting resident rooms between occupants. He kept to his early morning routine, hauling trash and cleaning litter from the yard, then drinking his coffee and reading the paper in the dining room. Ever the farm boy with chores to do, he took on more odd jobs around the house such as vacuuming the refrigerator and freezer coils, changing light bulbs, plunging clogged toilets, and cleaning the filters on the rooftop HVAC units. The children and I made Saturday morning pancakes, decorated holiday cookies, read aloud, and played Sorry! and Candyland. I took the occasional shift for a sick intern or PCA, washed down the hallways' wood trim to work off stress, and tried not to obsess too much about cleanliness and random concerns like whether we were using the dish sterilizer properly. I even began to enjoy planning and preparing for our community parties. The work was still intense and took most of my energies, but I felt a bit less anxious. I was falling in love with the community I had founded with such small understanding of how unprepared I'd been.

***

Kimberly had begun to mend fences with the sister caring for her six-year-old, Jamal. He'd contracted HIV/AIDS in utero or possibly during birth, having been born before studies proved that the drug AZT prevented transmission of the disease from mother to baby.

A woman already stigmatized with AIDS herself felt and was seen to be doubly guilty if she'd passed the disease to her baby. This guilt could be reason enough to succumb to addiction because drugs and alcohol temporarily masked the agony of having condemned a child to a sickly, pain-filled life and likely early death. In addition, relatives already frustrated with and hurt by the mother's drug use and disease could and often did use the baby's tragedy to further distance themselves from the mother.

This was Kimberly's story as well. Jamal was a small child who, because he had suffered precarious health his whole life, looked to be about five when he was actually seven. Kimberly had been only peripherally involved with her boy because her addiction to alcohol and crack had caused her sister to take the newborn from her. She'd done a beautiful job, from all appearances. Jamal seemed to be a happy and well-adjusted child.

When Kimberly first introduced him to me one Saturday afternoon, I was struck by how much he resembled his mother. On Jamal, the slight frame and impish features were sweetly appealing.

"Miss Carol, this my son, Jamal." Kimberly's face glowed. "He visiting while my sister shop."

The shy little boy shook my hand, and I saw Kimberly's own engaging smile on his face. I welcomed him to Miriam's House and watched him go up the stairs with Kimberly to her room.

I immersed myself in office work for a couple of hours, then wandered into the dining room for a break from typing policies and procedures. They were eating their afternoon meal, Kimberly's favorite sandwich, fried bologna and catsup.

"Hi, Jamal. Hi, Kimberly."

"Hey, Miss Carol." Kimberly turned cheerfully to Jamal. "Say hello to Miss Carol, Jamal." When he did, in his quiet voice, she looked at me with pride. "We eating dinner. Then we'll look at TV." She glanced at Jamal. "But I need a smoke after we eat. You okay going outside on the patio?"

The little boy nodded. Kimberly's face glowed. I picked up the Saturday paper and took a chair at the next table, peeping every once in a while over the top of the pages.

Jamal took small, thoughtful bites of his sandwich. Kimberly, long finished with hers, sat restlessly beside him, sneaking the occasional longing glance toward the window that looked out over the smokers' patio. More furtive yet were her quick, darting looks at Jamal. If their eyes met, she smiled and asked if he wanted more soda. He always said no.

"You done? You want another one?" Kimberly stood up and took his plate.

"No, ma'am." He looked at her, then away.

She turned to me, grinning widely. "Ain't he a polite boy, Miss Carol?"

I told the little guy how happy I was that he was with us and that I hoped he came back again. He smiled shyly, thanked me on Kimberly's prompt, and they left for the patio.

I wasn't on duty that night, so did not see him leave. But Heather said that, after her sister picked him up and drove away, Kimberly had stood looking after the car long after it had disappeared around the bend two blocks away. Then she took a patio chair and sat immobile, silent, not smoking, elbows on knees, head lowered between her bowed shoulders. Finally, she came indoors and went to her room.

She did not eat Sunday breakfast with us the next morning.

***

The period of time from spring to winter 1998 produced a lull. Later, we staff members would learn to tell one another to enjoy it now, take care of yourself and rest, because it will all change soon enough. But at that point we had not yet learned this wisdom, so the change, when it came, caught us by surprise. As I enjoyed the bit of quiet I could not know would end abruptly in December, I somehow thought we would go on together, these women, the staff, and Miriam's House, forever. Perhaps, in believing the worst times were over now that we were three years into being, I forgot that death and relapse and chaos could cycle back. I didn't know the not-worst times could still be very, very difficult. And, of course, we didn't know that Nickie, who had just moved in that May, was coming to the end of her life that December.

We didn't know until she was just about gone until our nurse, Kathy, who was with Nickie to help her dress, saw her suddenly collapse with a groan. Until Kathy raced up the hall shouting for me to dial 911 before running back to Nickie. What I remember is the look on Kathy's face as she knelt at Nickie's side, there on the floor in the bathroom, and that Kathy's eyes told me what we hadn't known.

I followed the ambulance to Howard Hospital, just a few blocks away. They pulled the stretcher out of the back of the vehicle, oxygen canister next to her and its mask over her face, one EMT scrambling alongside the stretcher performing CPR while the others rushed it indoors. I parked the car and ran into the ER, and they let me into the back without question once I said who I was and why I was there. But I was not allowed into the trauma unit, its curtain billowing outward with the hurried movements of multiple doctors and nurses, so I sat in a chair in the hallway, heart pounding. Twenty minutes later, a doctor sat down next to me to tell me, kindly and softly, that they had not been able to revive her.

"May I see her?"

"We need to clean her up first, but in about fifteen minutes, you can go in."

I told her we had a community of people who loved Nickie and asked if they could come to say good-bye. The doctor conferred with other ER staff, then returned to say we could have half an hour. I called Miriam's House to tell Tim and Angie. Then, seeing the activity in the trauma unit had ceased, I stepped in. But I couldn't control myself and was afraid that if I were heard, the permission to visit Nickie would be withdrawn. So I gave her a kiss on her cooling forehead and went outdoors to wait for my friends from Miriam's House, breathe deeply, and let the sun dry my cheeks.

Tim drove a group up in the van. The rest walked the few blocks. I recall standing with one hand resting on Nickie's foot, the other grasping Angie's hand. I tried to comfort the residents as they slowly entered the unit, stunned.

I don't know what happened after that, because I had to go to Nickie's father to tell him his daughter had died. I drove to the subsidized housing apartment building near Union Station where he lived, filled with dread, unsure of what to say and how to say it. I remember the smell of stale urine in the elevator. I remember wishing I had taken the stairs but then realizing they probably smelled worse and might be unsafe to boot. I remember the greasy feel of the air in the hallway, the dingy, indeterminate color of paint applied ages ago, the scuffed tile floor scattered with trash and cigarette butts, the yellowed ceiling above.

I waited long moments after knocking, listening to the shuffling sound of his approach, the wheeze of his breathing. Struggling for composure, I breathed deeply but choked on the stench. As Nickie's father opened the door I saw that the apartment was dark. Roaches scuttled away from the splash of hallway light on the kitchen floor and counters.

"Mr. Moore? My name is Carol. I work at Miriam's House, where your daughter, um, lives. May I come in?"

He opened the door farther and I walked in to the same smell as the hallway, only concentrated. Breathing through my mouth, I wrenched my mind away from the forlorn place and the disturbing thought of his living there. The elderly man shuffled and wheezed his way to the only chair in the tiny space.

"Who are you?" He had sat down heavily and now peered at me from rheumy eyes. I stood uneasily before him.

"I'm Carol." I tried again, "I work at Miriam's House with Nickie. I came to talk with you about her."

"Nickie?"

"Your daughter," I said faintly, quelling the rising nausea that now had less to do with the smell than it did with consuming sorrow that any human being had to live like this. I looked around the dingy apartment for a phone, a conviction growing in me that I would be unable to make him understand. Maybe I could call someone, a neighbor, to come over.

"Sir, I'm afraid I have bad news for you. I'm so very sorry. Sir?"

He had dropped his head and I noticed for the first time a fine trembling of all his body, as though within him sounded a tightly tuned cello string. I could not tell whether he'd understood what I'd said.

"Mr. Moore?"

"Nickie."

"Yes. Yes. I have come to tell you about Nickie. Your daughter." A fathomless river of suffering flooded ancient banks and boiled up through the soles of my feet.

He shook his head. "Nickie? Where is she?"

"Mr. Moore, do you have a friend living here? On this floor? Is there someone who can help us right now?"

"Herman. Next door."

And that is where my memory stops. I must have found Herman, he must have helped me find phone numbers for Mr. Moore's two sons. We must have called them, because I know I left with the assurance that a son was on his way. It would be a family member and not a stranger who would try to make this father understand that his only daughter was dead.

***

Something changed, or rather, tipped, in me after that. Perhaps it was that I needed just the one more experience of other lives. Perhaps I was finally ready. Because more than any other experience to that point, visiting Mr. Moore's smelly, roach-ridden apartment and seeing his illness and grief shoved me back against the bulwark of my assumptions. It made me assess the quality of my presence at Miriam's House. On the way home that day, I thought about how a woman who had just moved in would look around at the room we'd prepared for her and say it was the first time she'd ever had space to herself. She might talk about the moldy couch she'd been sleeping on in the basement of a relative's house because she had AIDS and wasn't allowed upstairs. She might mention the two-bedroom apartment she and her five siblings and parents had shared. Then she would close her door, alone, comfortable and safe for once. And I might get a bit sentimental as I went back to work, letting it go at that without much contemplating the implications. Until Mr. Moore.

Maybe it was the cumulative impact of Tamara and Kimberly and Little Mary. Maybe it was simply a learning moment. Because suddenly there I was, exposed to myself: judgmental, uncomprehending.

Who talks that way? I'd think as I passed the dining room and heard the raucous voices declaiming, often with loud disregard for "good" English, about private matters I'd been taught were not for public consumption. The volume, subject matter, and syntax were foreign and often distasteful to me.

My father, a journalism major in college and author of a couple of novels, had drilled his four kids on the finer points of grammar and usage, including liberal doses of commentary on our diction and pronunciation. He was a gentleman in the old-fashioned sense, gallant, polite, well-spoken. I only ever heard him curse once, a clipped *damn it* when he dropped a pancake on the floor. My mother is a reserved, dignified woman with strong ideas about what constitutes acceptable behavior. I had never heard her curse or make jokes other than those that were innocuous and silly. My parents were moral, upright, and conservative. They'd brought me up in way that was as far as it could get from life at Miriam's House.

And so, there were times when I judged the women wanting.

But then I saw Mr. Moore's pathetic apartment. I spent hours in the dining room at Miriam's House with our society's forgotten and derided ones. I celebrated holidays, sobriety anniversaries, birthdays, and GED graduations with them. We were together, cooking and eating meals, lighting memorial candles for our sisters who had died. We were together, popping popcorn, playing bingo, and preparing way too much food for community celebrations.

It was standing in Mr. Moore's smelly apartment and watching the roaches scatter, it was learning to rejoice in tinselly and overloaded Christmas trees. It was grasping Muriel's hand as she gasped her last, and keeping watch over lifeless bodies with the women lighting tea candles and sitting in prayer at my side. The cumulative effect of repeated dunking into the stream of life at Miriam's House put to shame my hidden assumptions of superiority. And I had to reject all familial and societal hierarchies relating to stature and language, education, class, and skin color.

This I had to go to Miriam's House to learn: in the most elemental moments of life, in those matters that draw from us our highest courage and most sorrowing despair, in the daily breaking of common bread, we are never other than one.

CHAPTER FOURTEEN

Much of life and work at Miriam's House was beyond my control, though that didn't keep me from casting about for something to obsess over. Once the smokers resigned themselves to using the front patio because they didn't want to pay fines, I guess I needed something else to do that helped me feel less at the mercy of ruthless fate. The handiest and most justifiable candidate was the dreaded roach.

I cannot stand roaches. Mice, I'm okay with. Spiders, thousand-leggers, bugs of whatever description, I might scream when I see them, but I'm not afraid to grab a tissue, sweep them up, and flush them away. But a roach gives me the creeps as does no other living creature, and I do not care who laughs at me about it. Really, I don't care that former residents continue to this day to find amusement in the story of The Roaches in the TV, nor that Donna, all these years later, collapsed with laughter the other day when I mentioned How I Made Doris Roar.

Both stories involve roaches and a television. Both involve a response that must have come from some primitive place deep in my brain over which I had no control. I will add with some pride, however, that my reaction in each instance was quick, decisive. I prefer to see this as indicative of my evolving leadership skills, rather than as an excuse for laughter at my expense.

The first incident, from summer 1998, occurred when I was watching TV one evening with a group of residents. To my extreme horror, I saw, running over the smiling face of a woman announcer on the screen, the silhouette of a roach. Then two. Then three.

I rocketed from my seat. "Oh my God, there's a roach, roaches, roaches inside the TV!"

I raced out of the room, paying no attention to the puzzled comments of a couple of the watchers. As I returned with a can of roach spray, one of them said, "Miss Carol, I think it's a commercial."

This observation had no braking effect on the forward momentum of my charge, arm extended, can aimed, finger on nozzle. I turned off the television and reached around to unplug it. "That was no commercial. Everybody out. *Out!* I'm gonna spray the hell out of this thing."

Another resident tried. "No, really, Carol, it was a commercial. Ain't no roaches up in there."

Too late. The women fled the room while I soaked the television in noxious spray.

"Die, vicious bastards!"

Congratulating myself on my quick reflexes, I barely registered the growing certainty, not to mention amusement, in the women's voices.

I spent a few days regularly checking the back of the television for roach carcasses. There were none, but I considered that insignificant. Until, that is, Kimberly raced up to me the next week, shouting. "Miss Carol, come quick. Them roaches!"

I sprinted to the TV room, battle-ready. There on the screen were the same silhouettes of scrambling roaches, the same woman with the same smile and the same lack of concern. I skidded to a halt.

"Oh."

Turning, I made what I hoped was a dignified retreat, pretending not to hear the shouts of laughter chasing me down the hall.

I had begun doing battle with roaches before I'd seen any, even before the residents had moved in. I'd hired an extermination company to make quarterly sweeps of the entire building. We also had a protocol for admitting new residents who, coming from overnight shelters and the like, tended to bring the vile things with them. Every box, bag, and appliance had to be checked by staff outside the front door before being brought indoors.

I was only vaguely aware of the moving-in activities on the afternoon that Doris came. I was stressed, glued to the computer trying to finish a grant application due the next day. These deadlines are written in stone. If you aren't prompt to the minute, your application will not be considered.

So all I could do that day was offer her a welcoming hug and make a swift observation of her grandmotherly face, modest stature, and reserved demeanor. Glad to close my door and settle in, blissfully ignorant of the Doris unrevealed to me in that quick meeting, I left the moving-in protocol to staff. Thank God for Donna, our new office manager, and the interns, who handled these things.

Donna's knock was so tentative that I realized I was hearing it for the second time. I called for her to come in, rubbing my tired eyes, fending off a feeling of doom. Donna never interrupted me unless it was important.

"Carol, I need to tell you something."

"Oh no."

"Yeah. Well, we just inspected Doris' things and found roaches in her TV."

Following close on her heels was the PCA on shift that afternoon. "Carol, you ain't want to get anywhere near that TV. Must be a thousand roaches up in there, hiding in the dark, ready to creep out at night."

Unsuccessfully suppressing a shudder and near desperation at the thought of my now-neglected grant application, I sort of exploded. "Where's the TV?"

"In front. I put it in a bag. Should we bomb it?"

"No. I'm pitching it." I swept past them and out the front door. Grabbing the tightly knotted bag, I hustled to the back of the building, heaved it and its repulsive occupants into the dumpster, then hurried back inside to wash my hands, return to my desk, and finish the application.

Or so I thought. Within minutes, Doris was at my office door. I don't actually know what she said. It's not faded memory after all these years, it's that she didn't speak, or even shout, so much as roar at me. That's the only way I can describe the shock wave of sound emanating from her mouth. The sole distinguishable word:

"*TELEVISION!*"

I would be frightened of a resident only one other time in all the years of my life at Miriam's House. In this instance, I didn't stop to think, not about my application, not about whether we might salvage the dumped TV. Gut fear alone spurred me into instant action. I fled, lingering only for the few seconds it took to mumble a hasty assurance.

An hour later I returned with a fourteen-inch color TV with remote control and asked Tim to set it up in Doris' room.

CHAPTER FIFTEEN

I can recall a time in my life when I was judgmental of addicts, if I thought about them at all. That was before I moved to Washington, DC, in 1990 to live and work at Samaritan Inns. And it was before I had learned that identifying the addict as the problem is, in itself, a problem.

**

A woman who has lived her addiction on city streets develops sensitive and acutely tuned antennae that she trains on anyone from whom she might get something: drugs, food, a favor, whatever. It's a sixth sense for sussing out precisely what that other person wants in order to deliver it, a means of assuring her own comfort or survival in the resulting exchange. Such were the women of Samaritan Inns: streetwise, intuitive, and acutely aware.

I moved into this group of women, still the people-pleasing, needy child, my thirty-five years notwithstanding. It was quite a crash: *I'll do what you want so you'll like me* meets *I'll pretend to like you to get you to do what I want.* And it took more than a couple of meetings with Clayton (*You're trying to get liked*) to make me figure out what the real problem was. In the end, I needed six months of bewilderment and Mary, a resident of the Inn with her infant son, John-John.

Mary was one resident at the Inn with whom I couldn't relate. She was mostly uncommunicative, and really gruff when she did communicate. She disliked me and made no concession to common courtesy when telling me so: "You a fake. I ain't trust you."

Not that her disdain would keep her from letting me help with her baby. During the slow afternoons of a duty shift, I would take the little boy to the Innkeeper kitchen where there was a rocking chair. Turning the stereo to my favorite classical music station and snuggling the sweetly sleeping baby on my chest, I'd rock, listen, and allow his innocent, nonjudging presence to soothe me.

Which was all the good it did me. "Why ain't you changed him?" she might say when I returned him. "Can't you tell he messed his diaper?"

My only response would be to cry alone in my room, flayed by her contempt. I just didn't get it. Couldn't she see that I'd completely changed my life in order to be here with her and the other women? Didn't that count for something? And how did it make me fake? And what about my ideals of being in service to the poor? How could I love and serve them if they were going to treat me like that?

We went on, the two of us, in mutual antipathy. Mary would storm up to me in a yellow sundress and with bare feet—in January—complaining about how cold the house was. She'd make sure to toss a gibe or two at me during weekly house meeting. I'd move to one side after opening the front door to let her in, the greeting dying on my lips as she brushed by with a grunt and a frown. I stayed away from the living room when I knew she was in there.

Had I known it would be like this when I decided to move to DC, I told myself, I never would have come.

After six months, Mary had a new complaint: "You don't never do urine screens. What's wrong with you?"

Part of my job was to do unannounced urine screens, at least three per month per woman. I hated it. I had to go into the teeny bathroom gloved and armed with sterile cup, watch her pull down her pants and sit on the toilet, hand her the cup and then stand there making sure she didn't cheat (substituting urine from another container, perhaps), while she sat there with her hand holding the cup between her thighs and trying to pee into it. How embarrassing. Some vestige of ancestral British reserve had left me with a prudish streak, so my face would redden and my hands tremble while I stood there beside the toilet. My solution had been to just stop doing them.

Mary was not going to let me get away with that.

"We be addicts. We'll live here happy that you don't never screen us and then go back out on the street because we ain't had to really be sober and we gonna use and then die. Well, I ain't wanna die. Do the screens."

She forced me to see myself through her eyes, bringing what Clayton had been trying to teach me into sharp focus. I had implemented a selfish pact: if I don't do the urine screens, they will like me. Except for Mary, the women were glad to pretend to like me so I wouldn't do the screens. All of us were complicit and considered it a small price to pay to get what we wanted. We addicts were enabling one another.

Here was a new world, a place so stern and uncompromising as to put me into the position of making an angry or reluctant woman pee into a cup while I stood and watched. A world in which actions that looked cold and even cruel—like turning away a pregnant woman on a wintery day—could actually be the most loving ones to take. Yet it was also so honest and self-aware as to allow for a stark realism, a pure kind of love: I love myself and you so much that I'm willing to face your anger and rejection. I choose to cease giving you what you want and what I want to give you. I'm even willing to do or say something distasteful in order that we stop deluding ourselves and live life with honesty.

I had to learn a new compassion, a different way of being in service, one that did not require the other to love or accept or treat me in a particular way in order for me to feel good about myself or my work. In this world I had to learn to serve without condition or hidden agenda, to be present to those around me in a way that was so very far from what I had called love, or from how I'd thought of service.

I had met the problem and she was not Mary, the homeless addict. She was me.

Anyone who has tried even to give up coffee in the morning, or whose doctor has instructed her to lose weight, knows that breaking an addiction is an act of monumental effort and determination. Really, it's all addiction—the indispensable morning cup of coffee, the cigarette break impossible to forgo, the one drink or glass of wine per day that slips unnoticed into three per day. Working obsessively to the detriment of personal relationship, shopping or eating in order to flee depression or fear, the need to be perfect or the best, the overwhelming desire to gain affection and approval. The accumulation of wealth, material goods, and status symbols beyond what is needed for survival and basic comfort and despite legions of people left hungry and unsheltered and our earth suffering irreparable damage.

Yes, we think, *but drug addicts and those alcoholics on the street are different. They're criminals, low-lifes. You can't equate them with me. I'm not in jail or homeless or dead.*

No, I cannot equate them. But that's not the point. It's about self-understanding leading to empathy. We can be honest with ourselves about our own addictions and notice our own reactions when asked to give them up. It may seem innocuous, that cup of coffee or two every morning or a growing interest in online gambling, but our emotional and physical responses to the suggestion of drinking less coffee or putting the computer away for a weekend are instructive. We know how hard it is to give up these everyday needs. Imagine how hard it is to give up crack, a similar but much more deadly struggle with an overwhelming need.

At Mary's instigation, my struggles with my addictive need to be liked became a leveling device that knocked me off my judgmental perch. These struggles lasted years, long into my time at Miriam's House. I still, to this day, catch myself upon occasion indulging in those old needy habits. How shall I judge the drug addict or the alcoholic?

***

Juanita, who lived at Miriam's House in 1999, told me the story of how she began using heroin. She could name the very moment. She was fourteen years old, watching a man shoot up heroin and begin to nod. He seemed oblivious of the people and noise and filth, and Juanita envied him.

"I wanted to go there, where he was, peaceful and no care about life or nothing."

Only fourteen? My dismay was raw, but she merely looked at me with those beautiful dark eyes and nodded, telling me,

"Ma would tie my hands behind my back, push me down on the floor, and beat me with the plug end of an electrical cord."

She asked, "You ever been beat like that?"

No, and it sounded unimaginable then, before I had heard so many similar life stories that it became all too horribly imaginable. The worst I got was a spanking over my dad's knee that didn't even leave a mark.

Juanita laughed. "That ain't a beating!"

She had just been beaten by her mother that day when the man on the back stairs shot up while she watched, a hot summer day with no school and nowhere to go to get away. The man, ragged and dirty as he was in that dingy stairwell, looked to her as though he'd been taken somewhere beautiful by that needle, somewhere better than this life of beatings and her mother's male friends hanging around, looking at her, wanting her.

"Do you know what men want girls to do?" Juanita described practices I wish I'd never heard. Yet what she was telling me were things that she had learned—no, not just learned, but experienced—as a young teen.

The summer I was fourteen, I spent every day at the company swimming pool where my dad worked. My mom would pack us a lunch, drop us off for swim team practice early in the morning, and then either pick us up in time for dinner at home or bring a picnic dinner to the pool. Those were my favorite days. Just after five o'clock, Dad would leave his office and come out to the picnic area, and we would eat together under a leafy tree with the sun low on the horizon and children's voices coming from the pool.

My special friends were other girls in my age group, five or six of us, together obsessing over our event times and helping one another through hard workouts. Once the competitive season ended, we took turns having sleepovers, during which we watched television, ate snacks, and gossiped about the urgent matters that absorb suburban teenage girls. One of the lifeguards taught a synchronized swimming class that we all took together, so the season culminated in a show that our parents and friends attended. Magical, endless summers, during which I learned to compete, excel at what I loved to do, and live joyfully into each sun-drenched moment.

All the while, Juanita was being tied up and beaten or handed over for the amusement of the men who "hung around." It was no stretch to realize that, had I been born into a situation such as Juanita's, I very likely would have ended up an addict on the street and, also like her, dead at thirty-three. None of us can survive trauma like that without finding ways to blot it out or get away. We seek the nodding bliss of a heroin high or something like it, each in our own way, because human minds and hearts are simply not equipped to stay present to such horror. We find ways to survive, only to have our strategies turn on us later, consuming us. Killing us.

CHAPTER SIXTEEN

Much of life at Miriam's House had settled into the familiarity of routine by the time 1999 began. The chaotic, seat-of-our-pants reactive mode of the first years had resolved into a calmer sense that we knew what we were doing and were doing it well. We had precedent for many of the circumstances we faced, and when there was no precedent we would say, not originally but accurately, *Never a dull moment at Miriam's House*. We had so far managed whatever tragic, silly, complicated, and always interesting events had happened in our community. Yet reassuring as this was, I continued to struggle with the question of whether I had stamina for the long haul. Oddly, and in opposition to the expectations with which I'd embarked on this venture, it was not the residents that made me wonder if I could stay. I was becoming much more comfortable with them. No, it was staff.

We held staff meetings on the ground floor in the efficiency apartment that at one time we'd thought would house live-in staff. We called it the lounge, but in the constant search for space we used it for any meeting that could not be held in an office, for napping on meal break, as a staging ground for parties upstairs, and for workshops and training sessions. The room had a quiet aspect, not fancy but pleasant, with its framed pictures on the walls, two windows, and comfortable couch. Not that a mere piece of furniture could make me comfortable there, at least not during staff meetings. The twelve of us sat ranged around the room in an oval that was meant to emphasize democracy. But I still had a difficult time hearing black women's voices as anything but angry. I continued to plead for agreement when open discussion was needed. And then there was the way three or four people would haggle over one subject, overtaking most meetings. Between my prejudices and insecurities and staff's lack of discipline, there was little of the democratic about these meetings.

In early January of 1999, the subject was Doris, who had begun to refuse to take her medications. One of the PCAs pursued the theme on which she and a couple others had already been harping for fifteen minutes.

"Kathy, Doris don't take her eleven o'clock meds, ever. Since I found that packet under her pillow, she just up and refuse them."

Kathy resolutely repeated what she'd said just a few minutes before, that we can't make Doris take her meds, that she had a right to refuse them. I looked at her sitting across the circle from me. In some ways, we were alike, white women often keyed up with nervous energy, brown eyes regarding the world attentively from angular faces with high cheekbones and determined jaws, and a sense of responsibility honed to the point of near morbid anxiety. But Kathy had a facility I had not yet mastered and therefore envied. She was able to separate what was her responsibility from what was not.

"We need to move on," she said.

Faye was not through. "But she's killing herself, Kathy. The medical professionals should be in control here. Why can't you talk to her?"

My heart sank. Now Faye had joined in, her brow creased with the emphatic scowl I cringed to see, her tone sounding aggressive and angry to me. And yet she was the one who insisted different departments not interfere with one another. I thought that, but was too chicken to say it aloud. I read her intervention as yet another baffling instance of what looked like arguing for the sake of arguing, a stance she took, it seemed to me, most particularly when she and I disagreed.

"I have been talking to her. What can I say that I'm not already saying?"

Kathy sounded frustrated. I felt it, too. This was just the latest in a series of such obsessive discussions that took time away from other, just as important, topics.

"So we gotta just watch her die?"

"No. No, we don't just watch her die, we keep doing what we're doing. It's not our job to force her or anyone to take medication, so we make sure the meds are ready for her, talk to her and support her . . ."

Kathy stopped. I looked around the circle and recognized the closed-face resistance that had silenced her. Faye trotted out her usual argument in such situations.

"She shouldn't have been allowed into Miriam's House in the first place. She's not mentally stable, and she's a dry drunk. Bad for the community."

That made me mad. "She does belong here. Doris is exactly who we're here for. We're not here to pick off the cream of the crop," I said heatedly. "We're here to serve women who have nowhere else to go, who have burned their bridges everywhere else."

"That isn't what I meant, Carol. You know that."

I didn't, but Faye and I were once again locked in a battle that neither of us possessed the power or will to change. Turning away from the fruitless fight, angry and tired of my struggles with Faye and this endless discussion, I had my own trotting out to do: I nagged at all of them.

I reminded them that it would actually be a violation of her civil rights to make her take the meds, at least here in DC, and she had the right to refuse medication or treatment, and it was no different from all the other issues we dealt with. "We can't *make* them stay sober, we can't *make* them give up that man we think is bad for them, we can't *make* them follow their budgets, and we can't *make* them see how they may be ruining their own health. When you think about it, we don't have much control at all over the women. What we have control over is the quality of our service, the extent of our compassion. That's all."

I knew I sounded hectoring but I had got up a head of steam and could not stop.

"You know all this. It's about our consistency, the quality of care, how well we care for them day after day. We have control over our own work, over what we provide and how we provide it. After that, the women decide."

Get over it, I wanted to say but didn't, though I was pretty sure everyone could read it in my voice or see it on my face.

Kathy said, "We don't get to choose. They choose for themselves. We don't get that choice."

Willing myself to ignore the fury on Faye's face and the frustration stabbing the air, I said, "Let's focus on the choices we do have and move on. We have other women to discuss here."

"They don't like the way you do that," Donna said to me later that afternoon. Donna, after substituting at the front desk for a couple of years, had become the full-time office manager recently, when Michelle, outdone by so much death, left and

Angela was promoted to take her place. "They feel like you're shutting them down."

"Yeah, I can tell. There's got to be a better way to get us out of that cycle of grinding on about one woman forever. I hate it. It doesn't get us anywhere."

Not only did it get us nowhere, it also meant that three or four staff members, usually the negative and contentious ones, did most of the talking most of the time. But I kept that thought to myself.

I went up to my apartment, reflecting on how staff meeting was the least-liked aspect of my week, and that personnel matters caused me more heartburn than any other part of my job. Staff meetings unnerved me; crises like a resident stuck in the elevator or a toilet overflowing did not. Dealing with Faye unnerved me; holding a dying woman did not. At the same time that I could moderate difficult discussions in house meeting, assuring each woman that her voice was heard and important, I responded angrily or defensively imposed my will when three or four people hijacked a staff meeting with their circular nattering.

What I wished to do was to listen, react, and speak from a calm center. How to keep anxiety from pushing me into ill-judged reactions? How to bring the decisive authority I exercised with Nickie, lying groaning and dying on the floor, to staff meeting disputes? If I had to leave Miriam's House, it would be due to my inability to resolve these conundrums.

I supposed I could just fire a few of them. I could make a strong case for lousy work performance on Ruby's part and insubordination on Faye's. I wasn't yet sure about Donna, who was learning well but was moody and picky about who she liked and didn't. And I'd belatedly become sure about one of the PCAs, who had been late for her shift a few times and once didn't show up at all.

"I should have fired her right then," I told David the next time we met. "I never should have kept her on after she didn't show, didn't call."

"Well, why didn't you?" asked David in his slightly ironic, humorous way.

I knew why he was asking that way. It seemed straightforward—you don't show, you don't keep the job. But truthfully, I hadn't thought of that, being more focused on getting her to see the impact her tardiness and absences had on her colleagues and on the women, trying to teach this woman who had worked little in her life how to hold down a job, how to be responsible. David asked whether I had ever fired anyone, making me respond somewhat spiritedly that of course I had fired people, like the children's program manager, and then there was that nurse who lasted only three weeks because she was fomenting discontent and rebellion with anyone who would listen to her.

David told me that during the early years at Joseph's House, they'd had a sort of triumvirate with three codirectors—himself, Sister Mary Daniel, and a nurse, Lois. When one of them was too close to the situation or too tired to deal with it, one or both of the others managed. "I don't know how you do this by yourself."

"Yeah, neither do I sometimes. Not to mention that I'm probably the worst person to have a job that entails being in conflict. I hate conflict. Anyway, when I think about firing Faye because she's really awful in staff meetings, it makes no sense. We need her. Faye is a really, really good addictions counselor."

Faye was loved by and effective with the women. With over 80 percent of our residents being recovering addicts, Faye's job was of urgent importance to women who—already saddled with the traumatic effects of poverty and low class status, abuse and cruelty, health problems like diabetes, high

blood pressure, and asthma, and, last but not least, AIDS—
were one step out the door from relapse into drug use and the
often violent life that went with it. I had sat through many a
Sunday meeting with Faye as she counseled a woman who had
used and come back to us ashamed and vulnerable, marveling
at her skill in combining straight talk about harsh reality with
compassionate understanding. Listening to and learning from
Faye was teaching me to respond better to residents. Was I to
fire her because she defied me at staff meetings and because I
didn't like her demeanor, only to lose the incalculable benefit
of her presence among and work with us?

Yet every time she opened her mouth, I wanted to argue
and, unable to stop myself, did, despite being far outclassed. I
had grown up in a family that did not acknowledge anger per
se, and so I argued ineffectively. Fights with my sisters had usually been screaming matches that ended after scant seconds
with combatants sulking behind slammed doors. They had not
prepared me for the kind of disputes familiar to black women
raised on the streets of DC. So I was easily intimidated, invari-
ably ending up on the defensive and quickly silenced. Faye's
was an offensive game. In any confrontation between her and
me, the smart money was on Faye.

"The place would go up in flames if I got rid of Faye, so I
keep her on even though we fight at every turn."

I told David I really didn't believe Faye when she said she
wasn't angry, just passionate. To me, it looked and sounded
like anger, so I would react with anger and get defensive.
Constructive communication had no chance.

David told me that after he'd lived in DC for a while, he
started to see that surviving in the city meant growing a kind
of thick skin he realized he'd never grow because life had never
forced him to. That, and staying on the attack, being aggressive

in order not to lose a fight, or if you did lose, not being completely overwhelmed and looking weak or vulnerable.

"It's quite an accomplishment to survive childhood if you're black and living in DC, when you think about it. My guess is that it takes an impressive amount of courage and energy to live like that, a certain *kind* of courage and energy. You don't unlearn all that just because you get a job."

And there I was, no good at confrontation unless I felt I was absolutely in the right, and even then no match for most of my staff. I was sure they knew that. "I'll bet they think I'm a wimp. A pushover."

And Faye was only the most notable of the people I was straining to understand and handle.

Donna's moods swung unpredictably from warm and friendly to icy and distant, fluctuations signaled by her large, expressive eyes. A good mood meant we would joke around a bit, offer to answer phones so the other could take a break, and cooperate with easy humor on one of the many tasks we handled together. A bad mood meant she would barely greet me and look away as I was speaking to her, making our collaborations strained and unfriendly. Although she was careful not to let me see it, I found out after too long a time that she was at least as unfriendly, if not worse, to others to whom she had taken a disliking. Yet she was turning into a most valuable staff member. She learned the office and building systems well enough to manage emergencies when Tim and I were not around. She walked the various inspectors around the building, usually charming them so that a tour that had begun with a stern-faced official ended with a smiling guy who sat in her office to joke and chat for a while. She kept the storeroom neat and stocked with supplies. Any children in the house magically obeyed her, and all it took was a look. They also loved to sit in her office and do their homework or perform some small task she gave them. She was the person on whom I could most rely when I rushed away to attend to a disaster in the house or an urgent call from a hospital. It seldom happened that resident confrontations turned physical, but for some reason two of them did in front of Donna's office. She handled the altercations with an authority and stature I could only dream of having. And many residents loved her. They would sit in the chair near her desk and stay for hours, sometimes chatting but mostly just being with her.

Then there was Ruby, a PCA who was herself one misfortune away from qualifying as a resident, and for whom I had an affection that blinded me to the larger effects on the community of her inconsistent work ethic, nonexistent professional boundaries, and penchant for spreading gossip. I was caught in a back-and-forth cycle with her, in which she'd gradually let her behavior and work deteriorate until I called for some sort of sanction like a warning or a suspension, after which she'd improve. For a while. Yet even being aware of that cycle was not helping me get out of it.

I wanted to be fair to people whose lives had been so much more difficult than mine, whose worldly education had come at the expense of their self-esteem and sense of position in our society. This desire to be fair kept me in dialogue, trying to instill better work habits, stressing the necessity of reliability and good community relationships, being satisfied with evidence of sincere effort and ability to grow. It was hard work for me. I mostly just wanted everyone to get along, do what they were supposed to do, and make my job easier.

Additionally, the porous membrane serving as inadequate protection for my feelings ensured I took personally the negativity and complaining that are part of every workplace. Easily hurt, I tried to hide my feelings, in part because I could see that the snarling of communication was due time and time again to

my impatience with modes of expression unfamiliar to me. Or
to my insistence that my way was the best way.

Another aspect of the fairness matter had to do with the
fact that black staff were, with only two exceptions over seven-
teen years, the ones with whom I contended. If I fired everyone who fought with me, or needed to learn how to act more
professionally, or with whom I had style differences, I would
have scoured the black personnel roster almost to the bone.
Then the temptation would have been to fill it with white, middle-class people who looked, acted, and thought a lot like me
while looking, acting, and thinking nothing like the women we
served.

Somehow, somewhere, I had to find a balance. I needed to
find a way to be understanding and aware of the cultural, educational, and economic differences of our lives while making
sure staff worked hard and served the residents well. Because
there was only one bottom line: the women must get the best
we could give them.

During our weekend walks downtown, I'd often chew
over these seemingly intractable problems with Tim. He was
patient and helpful in these conversations that took on their
own pattern.

"It's not about guilt," I might say, referring to my sense of
fairness. "I mean, it's not about feeling guilty because of black/
white history in this country. But I do feel and see and hate its
effects, past and present. Besides, when someone raises it, as
in *I don't have to feel guilty for something that happened long
before I was born*, it seems to come more out of their unwillingness to admit to continuing inequalities than it does from
wanting to make things better. Status quo is always more
comfortable."

Tim would nod. He was the one who'd introduced me to
the concept of white privilege: we white people benefit from a

system so biased toward us that we can't see it, yet instinctively don't want anything to change in case our benefits go away.

But even knowing and feeling passionate about all that, when it came to staff relations, part of me just wanted to stamp my feet and pitch a fit, as in *Why the hell doesn't everyone just shut up and do their jobs?* Or, more accurately, *Why can't everyone just be nice to me and do exactly what I want?* Although it wasn't just about me, either—I wanted to figure out a way to have good, consistent staff discipline *and* fairness around racial and educational inequalities *and* really good care for the women. Which was the most important thing, really. Good care for the women.

One Saturday Tim slowed and looked at me, asking if that weren't the easier problem to solve, that what would make things really bad for me would be if I were afraid of death, or disliked hanging out in the dining room, or dreaded writing procedures and running the organization. I didn't get it. He tried again.

"You have the things that can't be learned. Compassion, enthusiasm, love for the work, desire to improve, and self-awareness. You just need better leadership skills, learning how to manage and supervise people. That stuff can be taught. Plus, you're in a good place for it, with all the training and classes in DC."

Within a week I'd found a professional development organization that was, in cooperation with Georgetown University, creating a pilot program for nonprofit executive directors. My board of directors approved the expense, and I registered to begin the six-month leadership-training course in November. Even just knowing help was near improved my confidence.

I'd been ploughing through my days with head down and nose pressed to my work, so myopically focused on the burden of responsibility and the problems with my board of directors that I was missing important parts of Miriam's House life. I felt heavy, awkward, clumsy. Yet I so wanted to feel light underneath the cares of my job. I tried to remind myself to lift my head, take a deep breath, and remember the horizon was far beyond, beckoning, and maybe even freeing.

CHAPTER SEVENTEEN

We named it the Kimberly Policy because we wrote it specifically for her. As it turned out, we would have to invoke it for no other resident. It served its purpose just once: to get a healthy and stable Kimberly to move out so that her room was freed up for someone who was really ill and struggling.

Kimberly—drunken object of police attention two times that we knew of, flouter of rules and defier of even minor expectations—had decided in mid-1998, for reasons unknowable to us, to work her program. By the end of that year she was stable in her community relations, improved in health, and almost one year sober. She had successfully turned away from "the lifestyle," as the residents termed it, which was quite an achievement. We were justifiably proud of Kimberly, partly in view of all we had gone through with her, but most especially because of the strength and determination required of her to make such a change. We decided that Angie and Faye would begin to talk with her about moving out into independent living, a goal we were sure she would embrace with the same enthusiasm that others had.

Once again, we had failed to take into account the Kimberly we had known, loved, and fought for three years.

"Ain't going nowhere. Staying here."

"Yeah, that's what Angie told me you said to her."

I had caught up with Kimberly on one of her restless journeys through the house the evening after Angie reported her heels-dug-in reaction to the idea of moving out. I was determined to let her go only after making a point or two, resolutely ignoring the unsubtle glances she directed toward the front door and the smokers' patio. I reminded her that she was stable, doing well after an almost miraculous turnaround, and that she could always come back, like Crystal did after that surgery, if she needed us temporarily. And she would feel so good about herself as she took on more responsibilities and become more independent.

"But I ain't wanna leave, Carol. I'd be dead by now if it wasn't for Miriam's House. I'm staying."

Truthfully, part of me didn't want her to leave, and I told her so. But then I reminded her how sick she'd been when she first came to us, that she couldn't stay sober and was thin as a rail, popping in and out of the hospital. "There are women like that out there now who need your room. They should get the chance you've had. Besides, remember how you hate the rules? Hate curfew? Hate giving up a urine screen?"

Kimberly, with the gruff charm I loved, laughed her acknowledgment of the irony, but remained steadfast. Eventually we took matters into our own hands, all the while trying to get her to see the value of self-sufficiency. Angie found her a room at Shalom House, a single-room-occupancy residence in Northeast DC, where she would have an added measure of independence but enough supervision to help her stay focused and sober.

Thankfully for all of us, Kimberly did become positive about the move once she visited Shalom House, met some of the residents, and saw her room. Meanwhile, I wrote the policy that was thereafter presented to each new resident. It told them that when they became stable we would help them find another place to live in order to free up their room for someone who needed it more. No other woman ever required our citing it.

I had been honest about not wanting Kimberly to go. I never really wanted a resident to leave because the leaving always tore a hole in the fabric of our community. Yet I loved the fact of these strong women; the heart needed to stay sober and follow all the medical regimens and let go of dysfunctional habits and deal with faltering mental health. I loved living and working in a place where that could happen. I loved being part of the process. So if their leaving was the outcome of all that I loved, then I might as well embrace it, however difficult it was.

By January 1999 we'd celebrated the moving on of several women: Paula, to an apartment and hair-styling school; Norah, to an apartment and volunteer work sharing wisdom about AIDS and recovery; and another who married and then adopted her grandchild after her daughter died. Kimberly's moving-out party that month followed the traditions already established, with housewarming gifts from Miriam's House and residents, a community meal followed by sharing our good-byes and well-wishes, and then the drive to the new place in a van packed with bags and boxes.

On the evening of Kimberly's party, I sat in the dining room, remembering the place as it had been in 1995 during construction, and recalling Kimberly as she'd been when she first came to us. I looked around at the chattering groups and marveled. The women were making this place a home. I'd had that thought many times, but on that night I realized my feelings of dismayed superiority had finally melted away. Feeling humbled and more than slightly ashamed, I let myself take in the rhythm and intent of their speech, and thought mine seemed pallid and evasive in comparison.

***

If the main purpose of the spoken word is to communicate, these women were communicating with a stripped-to-the-essence, naked forthrightness that contained its own searing beauty. Perhaps I'd cringed early on at the cursing and the subject matter, but it put my reticence to shame. The women opened a window on the devastating reality of lives very different from mine. Perhaps I knew a more elegant way to speak, but their speech—with its intimation of endurance and what had been endured—scraped me raw. I can imagine my face betrayed some of my thoughts, and my silence gave me away. And perhaps many of the women did ease up on angry language and censor subject matter when I was around. Most of them during my fourteen years at Miriam's House wouldn't say the word *bitch* in conversation if I were nearby. They'd say *B* instead, as in *"She called me a B, Miss Carol."*

It had taken these years until I was able to listen beyond the curse words and ungrammatical phrases, the anger and sketchy subjects. I wanted to relate at a deeper level than the grammatical, the syntactical, and the socially acceptable. As I lay aside my snobbery and prudery in order to really listen, I began to hear musicality, rhythm, and expressiveness in what I'd censured. Because dancing within those qualities was honesty: honesty that mocked the superficial niceties and polite nothings I habitually spouted, honesty the likes of which I had never before encountered. This was the grammar of women excoriated by circumstances not of their choosing and by the choosing they had done in order to survive. This was the syntax of the recovering addict who had all but killed herself with dishonesty and excess and denial and fear and who knew that unpolished reality was her salvation.

Once I began to hear it differently, the women's language so compelled me that I would mimic it without knowing, just as I might the accent and syntax of a visitor from England. I even came to the point of taking their example a little too freely. And I never realized I'd made the adjustment until I unconsciously employed Miriam's House language or subject matter in one or two e-mails or conversations with family members. In their bemused reactions, I recognized my own early responses to the women of Miriam's House. But for now, listening in a new way, all I could think about was how much I had to learn from my new community, my new family.

***

The sharing usually took place between dinner and dessert, which had the advantage of allowing the smokers to go outside to the patio, have their cigarette, and come back in as the sharing began. And, not incidentally, avoid altogether the cleanup activities between dinner and dessert.

"Kimberly, you been a inspiration to me. You kept clean even when Kyle was gone, you kept focused, and you didn't relapse. I was watching you 'cause I was scared for you. Remember that talk we had? Here in the kitchen?"

"I ain't liked you at first, Kim. You ain't liked me. But we be friends now. And all that damned fried bologna! You better learn to cook something else, girl, you'll make yourself sick. But I wish you the best in your new place."

"I'll miss you, Kimberly, I really will. Won't be the same around here without you."

"Kimberly, I just got here so I don't know you real well. But I hope you do great in your new place."

"I'm gonna miss them horror movies on the weekend. I'm gonna miss your laugh and how excited you get when you hit the numbers, and seeing little Jamal here sometimes."

"I just think about that blond hair. Girl, I'm so glad you let that grow out. Don't do nothing crazy like that now, don't go out there and fuck up. And come back to visit, you hear?"

"Kimberly, stay strong. Stay home. Don't fuck up. Ain't nothing out there you need. Stay close to the staff at Shalom. Go to meetings. Get a sponsor, stop fooling around with that. You need a sponsor now that you ain't here no more. And good luck."

CHAPTER EIGHTEEN

It wasn't so much Alyssa's skeletal limbs that shocked me every time I looked at her, as she carried those 110 pounds on her five-foot-eight frame with a certain strange grace. This was toward the end of those long and tragic years when almost everyone with AIDS sickened, diminished horribly, and died a lingering death. The change from death sentence to chronic illness had already begun for others. But for so many of our women it had come too late, or they'd been too busy taking care of others to take care of themselves, or the new drugs were too toxic, or bodies already ravaged by poverty, poor health care, and multiple forms of abuse could not tolerate them. So it was for Alyssa. The ravages of AIDS on Alyssa's young body—she was just twenty-four in early 1999—declared themselves most emphatically on her face, with its sunken cheeks outlining the shape of jaw and teeth, its skin stretched tight over high, prominent cheekbones, and in the eyes an expression I have only ever seen in the dying.

I didn't know Alyssa very well, at least not until she was bed bound. She was with us only five short months before she died, and was younger than all of us except one other resident, Brianna. Yet some vivid memories remain, like her pride in offering suggestions for improvements and in seeing them implemented, how she loved gospel music and Sundays at her church, the way she looked as she and Brianna headed out on one of their day-long excursions. And how she died.

She usually made her suggestions at house meeting, during the time when residents shared comments, criticisms, and compliments.

"Mr. Tim, why don't you put up something so we have cups at the water purifiers? You should get those long containers that the cups come out of the bottom, paper cups, it would be better for us."

"We need one of them tall cigarette ash can things out on the front patio. Them little ash trays on the table aren't big enough and they make a mess. And they smell."

During the one winter Alyssa was with us, and after she became ill enough that traveling by Metro was too taxing, she asked us to make sure she got to church every Sunday. I began driving her there after Sunday breakfast, and Faye picked her up midafternoon. I'd pull up to the side entrance, drag her wheelchair out from the back of the van, turn around, and find a crowd of church members eager to assist her from her seat and into the chair. Here was one church that made no judgment about AIDS, and the look on Alyssa's gaunt face was gift indeed.

One morning, I startled Alyssa as she came out her door and almost bumped into me.

"Miss Carol, what are you doing there? Scared me."

"I'm sorry. It's just that I love hearing your music, and sometimes I stop on my way down to the office. You know, to borrow a bit of peace before the confusion starts."

"Oh, well, go ahead. I put it on every morning and pray."
She walked down the hall to the shower and I, down the stairs
to my office.

Alyssa and Brianna, on days when they had no appointments or meetings, would go out together for a day of visiting, shopping, and best of all, a burger-and-shake lunch at
Checkers. The two of them, giggling, hurrying impatiently past
us stodgy oldsters toward the world outside, bundled against
the cold, bursting out the front door and not to be seen again
until curfew, reminded me strongly of my nieces, of life and
future and youthful joy in just being. Except that Alyssa had a
deadly disease. Except that when she was twelve, her mother,
who needed money to pay the drug man, had put Alyssa on the
street as a prostitute.

One might expect that Alyssa would be bitter, having
been betrayed by the person whose trustworthiness was most
urgently necessary to her young life. She was not. One might
expect that Alyssa would be reclusive, the dying she was under-
going engraved upon her face. She was not. And this is what
stays with me about Alyssa, that in her was no anger, no hiding
from the world, no cynicism. She was street smart, of course,
and could give as good as she got, which, at Miriam's House,
meant she had a sharp tongue and a talent for the swift retort
expressed in colorful language. But I never heard her say anything negative about her mother. Nor did she stop trying to see
her—not when they made plans that her mother didn't keep,
not when her mother reneged on her promised attendance at
Alyssa's birthday party in May.

On a day that turned out to be just two weeks before her
death, Alyssa tried again.

"It's spring, it's warmer. I'll be fine."

"Well, it's only May, and the weather can change quickly."

I had come into the nurse's office on some errand, heard the tense exchange, and saw the determination on Alyssa's face, the hesitation on Kathy's. Alyssa told me that she wanted to go visit her mom. At home. "Someone can drive me in the van. It's not even as far as church, just over the bridge in Southeast."

Like Kathy, I hesitated. The story of Alyssa's life was appalling and her current situation only nominally better in that she was safe and comfortable. Her mother had never once adhered to any commitment to visit her daughter, despite Alyssa's regular invitations. I still felt my useless rage of the night of the birthday party when I found Alyssa sitting alone in her wheelchair in the front hall, staring out into the darkening evening, waiting. Finally, we'd persuaded her to come to the dining room because the food was getting cold and the party needed to start.

But now the expression on Alyssa's wasted face was so hopeful that I softened. I told her that if she wanted to go, we would work it out. Angie could call her mother. Jan and Sarah, our newest intern, could drive her over and pick her up a few hours later. "Is that okay?"

"Yeah. But I can call my mom."

"Well, let Angie call, too. Just to make everything really clear."

It would only be a cruelty to remind Alyssa about her birthday party and all the other times her mother had let her down. I left the office because I wanted to get to Angie before she was gone for the day and because I was afraid to say anything more in front of Alyssa.

Downstairs in her office, Angie and I agonized. It seemed too cruel for words, the mother who never showed up despite Alyssa's incessant attempts to get her attention. Why the hell couldn't that woman make one simple gesture for her daughter? And what made us think she'd come through this time? For all we had seen, she had never come through, ever.

"I know, Angie, but you should have seen the look on Alyssa's face. I couldn't argue, I just couldn't. What was I supposed to do, convince her that her mother won't show?"

"It's like a last wish," said Angie softly.

So Angie, Jan, and Sarah worked quickly to arrange the trip. We were not sure how much longer Alyssa would be strong enough to go out of the house. She was in hospice care and already dividing her day between wheelchair and bed, mostly reliant upon the PCAs and Kathy for bathing, dressing, and cooking. With no sense that this was going to work out, we watched as Jan and Sarah loaded the wheelchair into the back of the van and helped Alyssa in.

Dismay set in hard when they returned and Jan said it had looked as though no one was home.

"She insisted we leave her there. She said she had a key. All we could do was say we'd be back at four o'clock. We'll leave early to pick her up, just in case."

And a good thing they did leave early, because Alyssa's mother was not at home and had never come home and Alyssa had lied about having a key.

They found Alyssa still in front of the house, but didn't know until she told them on the ride home that she'd been outdoors the whole time. And there was a group around her, so they thought she'd met up with friends and that it had been a good visit. They were happy for her and relieved. But then, as they got out of the van and approached, they saw the kids gathered around Alyssa were somber. They heard weeping.

Alyssa, sitting outdoors for three hours in the community of her childhood and teen years, had attracted the attention of neighbors. Gradually, high school friends had gathered. I could only imagine what they felt upon seeing a skeleton in the wheelchair instead of the Alyssa they remembered.

"It was awful. That little shabby house with its dirt yard." Jan shook as she spoke. Alyssa's life had been so hard and yet she wanted to go back, wanted to see that woman (neither Jan nor I could refer to her as anything but "that woman"), who'd shoved her out on the street and then smoked up the money she earned. It made Alyssa's love seem both noble and pathetic. Seeing her there, stuck in that straggly place, had reminded Jan of her own youth on a Nebraska farm under an endless sky. The contrast had done her in.

They brought Alyssa home. She asked to go to bed. Within a week, the hospice nurse told us death was near.

My final memories of Alyssa are of her asking and then, after speech was not possible, reaching for, her mother. At her bedside, I tried to hide my anger at the woman who had put Alyssa into this bed with this horrid disease that brought this death so young.

In Alyssa's small, cozy room that was the first of her own and last of her life, we made her final days as cheerful as we could. Kathy and the PCAs comforted and bathed her, changed the bed sheets, spruced up the room with photos, cards and stuffed animals, and kept her clean. I put the chart outside the door and the "In the Event of Death" folder on the table in my office, all notification forms completed. Staff and residents alike visited often and kept the gospel music playing. We sat with her, read to her, relayed house gossip. We tried to be diplomatic when she asked for her mother, unwilling to say that all our messages about Alyssa's deterioration had gone unanswered.

Being Alyssa, she determined to take charge of the matter herself. She would insist that someone dial the phone for her, dictating the number in her quavering voice because her fingers were too weak and her hands too shaky for her to press the phone buttons. When, inevitably, the answering machine came on, Alyssa left a message. She always left a message. She never got a call back.

She did not stop asking us to dial until she ceased speaking altogether.

At eleven o'clock on that final night, I opened the door to Alyssa's room, ready to begin my vigil. But instead of the quiet scene I expected, I saw Jan sitting on the bed beside an agitated Alyssa, whose impossibly thin body somehow still had the strength to struggle wildly. Neither Jan nor Alyssa spoke. I put down my mug of tea and got to the other side of the bed as quickly as I could.

"What's she doing?"

We sprawled across the bed and attempted to control the flailing arms.

"She's not talking, just seems to be trying to get out of the bed."

Further conversation was impossible. Somehow we got her quiet, lying back, only her eyes darting about the room and her hands plucking at the sheet we'd pulled up around her. Jan looked plain worn out, as though she had reached the limits of her stamina for this dying.

"I'll stay with her. Go get some rest. You look done in. And thank you, thank you."

After Jan left, I called hospice. The nurse on call instructed us to give Alyssa one of the antianxiety medications left with us for just such situations. The PCA on night shift helped me find the medication, and I placed it under Alyssa's tongue. Then we settled into the familiar routine developed over so many other nighttime vigils, the PCA leaving the room for the other responsibilities of her shift while I remained. Every hour or so, she'd come in to check on us, often giving me a short break to stretch my legs or go to my apartment to make a cup of tea.

I found little things to do, as much to keep myself awake as to comfort my dying friend. Sometimes reading, sometimes humming one of her beloved gospel songs, sometimes massaging sweet-smelling lotion onto rough, dry skin, often completely quiet. In that somber and timeless space with the two of us suspended in the unknowable, we waited.

Toward two o'clock, Alyssa, perhaps as the medication wore off, began shifting in the bed with enough energy that the sheets became wound around her torso. I called for the PCA as, silent and again with that surprising strength, Alyssa was suddenly upright in bed and extending emaciated arms as though offering—or asking for—a hug. Just as we were deciding to call hospice again, Alyssa spoke. We turned to her in disbelief.

"Ice cream. I want ice cream."

"You stay, I'll go for it." she sped from the room.

Perhaps making the request had taken all she had, for Alyssa lay back, saying nothing more. She turned her head, her eyes flickered. Watching? Waiting?

The PCA returned with a small dish of the ice cream left over from Alyssa's twenty-fifth birthday party. She carefully placed a very small amount on Alyssa's tongue. We were afraid she would choke but wanted her at least to enjoy its cool sweetness. And it did seem to help, because she lay back, eyes open but no longer darting about, arms resting at her sides. After a few minutes, seeing Alyssa was quiet once more, the PCA left. Alyssa lay still a while.

When she finally moved, she grabbed my hands so quickly that she was clutching me before I could respond and she said, "Hold me."

So strong was her grasp I could not shift my position in the chair by her bed. I simply held on as tightly as I could. I whispered to her. *I'm here. I'm here.*

After several moments, she said, "Let me go." We released our grip on each other. I shifted from the chair *it's okay, all is well* to sit on the bed beside her and facing her *it's okay, you are doing great, you are strong, you are so beautiful.*

She struggled upright, drawing me in close for a hug of desperate strength. She whispered, and it was steady and strong and knowing. "I have to go."

Yes, dear one, it's all right, you are doing so well and her arms relaxed *you are so beautiful, you're doing great, all will be well* as I cradled the back of her head and neck in my hand *go, if it's time to go, God is waiting* and gently I laid Alyssa down *God loves you* slipping my hand out from behind her neck, smoothing the sheets around her body, angling my head so that the tears would not fall on her face *we all love you.*

And she reached out no more, she said no more, she only bit and gulped *we love you* and clenched and grimaced, cords on her neck straining, fighting for *go to God* every breath, breath after breath after breath until the last breath *we all love you* and even then biting and stretching and gulping in a slow diminuendo *God loves you* that ended in a silently defiant, almost imperceptible *we love you* lift of her chin.

When on that dark morning Alyssa finally stopped fighting, when I had stopped sobbing, all I could think was that she'd had only one taste of the ice cream now melting in the dish on the table by her bed.

***

After I bathed her face, combed her hair, straightened her limbs and once more smoothed the sheets about her, I called the PCA, who tearfully sat down by the bed to keep watch a while. Then I went to my office for the "In the Event of Death" folder in which I had my list of residents who wanted to be awakened if Alyssa died at night and staff members who wished to be called and told.

And so I scuffed slowly through the sleeping house, tapping on certain doors and whispering to sleepy residents who had arisen at my knock already knowing why I was there, and who hugged me and asked, also whispering, if I was okay.

"You got the little candles in there? I want to light a little candle for her."

"She's in a better place, no more suffering. Don't be upset, Miss Carol, she be better off now."

"I'll wake up Brianna. She ain't want no one to tell her but me."

"Where Rita? She in there with her? I'll go see her, she'll be upset about this."

"You gonna call staff now? You know not to call Donna, right? She ain't want to know at night, she want to know when she get here in the morning and can be with all of us."

"I can't go in there now, I can't do it. I'll stay in my room and pray. Light a little candle for me."

Alyssa's body, barely lifting the clean, white sheet enshrouding it, received us as we sat with her in the familiar ritual. Lighting small tea candles from the white pillar candle on the table next to her body, we kept silence in the unsteady light.

Perhaps hell is here on earth for those who so utterly destroy a young person. I cannot know what awfulness must have occurred in Alyssa's mother's own life, or in that of the men who so cruelly used her, or even what demons they let drive them, that they could do this to a child. I have lit many tea candles, and by their faltering light I have sat watch over many women. Yet only once did I do so with anger-scalded grief, and that was when I sat watch over Alyssa.

***

Alyssa's life had left her with no one who could arrange or pay for a funeral. Certainly her mother was no more prepared to be present to her daughter in death than she had been in life. By dint of much phone calling and with the help of community activist Earline Budd, we found a funeral home that took Alyssa as a charity case, charging nothing as long as we were willing to wait until they had time to fit her in. So it was several weeks instead of the usual five or six days until we could hold her funeral. But that seemed a small matter compared to the morticians' generosity.

The line to view Alyssa in the open casket at the front of the church moved unusually quickly. People were stopping at the casket and turning away almost immediately. I didn't realize why until I stood there and looked down. Alyssa's face had a sallow, almost yellow, hue. The padding used to plump her cheeks was visible under her face's too-thin skin and her cheekbones seemed razor sharp. Her lips were forced into a rigorous grin. Later I wondered if the funeral home, located in an affluent part of the city, had ever prepared a black woman before, or maybe had spent too little time preparing this body for which they were getting no payment. But this was our final memory of Alyssa, and it held us in grief far beyond our usual mourning period.

That, and her mother didn't show up.

***

After Alyssa died in May of 1999, I needed to slow down, to get out of the city with its constant motion and noise and concrete and buildings. I had spent many weekends in retreat at Dayspring, the Church of the Saviour's retreat center, and always returned refreshed, but wanted to go farther away this time. I found a place just outside of Philadelphia in a lovely setting with woods and deer so accustomed to human presence they would allow me to come within a few feet of them before bounding off.

But four days could not possibly be long enough to effect much change in what was bred-in-the-bone, that driven, nervous style that so often interfered with my ability to be present to my little community. On the train returning to DC, and already becoming anxious again, I regretted that the retreat had not seemed to slow me down much. Too soon, however, I had something bigger to regret. By the second morning after my return I felt lousy with chills and aches. That afternoon, I noticed two red spots, one on my abdomen and one on my upper thigh. By the time the spots had developed into the classic bull's-eye rash of Lyme disease, I was at the ER with a smashing headache and a high fever.

For the first weeks, Tim came up from the office every couple of hours to see how I was doing and make me a cup of tea or change the radio station. Once the headaches subsided after about four weeks, I read a lot of books, napped often, and counted it a triumph when I could get to the bathroom without crawling.

I had slowed down.

After six weeks or so, I managed an hour in the office every morning, responding to phone messages, reading e-mails, and catching up with the women. From late August through October, that hour gradually increased to a full day. Not until after the first of the year did I get my old energy back, although I had improved enough to begin my leadership course in November. A bit shakily I faced the 1999 holiday season that, this year, included bonding with Faye over a bit of holiday larceny.

***

Tim and I had learned early on to create good boundaries because we lived where we worked and because the nature of the community—vulnerable, unpredictable, and tending, without great vigilance, to the unstable—required we protect ourselves. We agreed on a time limit if work matters needed to be discussed in the apartment. We asked residents and staff not to raise business or community matters when we were off. We'd begun arranging long weekends away every three or four months. As we added to the policies and procedures manual, staff had authority to solve problems without resorting to us. I designated Sundays as my quiet day. Of all these practices, the one that the community most honored was my Sunday practice, and after breakfast was over they did everything they could not to bother me. When they did have to call me, it would be for a good reason, such as the Sunday Faye phoned to say she was about to be arrested and would I help.

"Carol, please tell this man I'm a staff member at Miriam's House."

"Where are you? What are you talking about?"

"I'm at the Ames store, Fourth and Rhode Island. They think I was shoplifting with Latrice. They think I was driving the getaway car." Her voice shook.

"I don't . . . getaway car?"

"Yes, yes, and they're trying to arrest me. Just please, just talk to this man!"

Fortunately, the security guard was calmer than Faye and more lucid than me.

"Ma'am, we have Faye Powell here with Ms. Meckel, who is detained for shoplifting. Ms. Powell states she's is a staff member at Miriam's House, but we found her in the parking lot in a maroon van and so we have her as an accomplice. Looks a lot like she was driving the getaway vehicle."

That steadied my shaken attention. "Sir, I can assure you that Ms. Powell is a longtime and trusted member of my staff. She has permission to take the residents out on Sundays during her shift. She's not driving a getaway vehicle. I promise you she didn't know what was going on inside your store."

The security guard believed us. He released Faye, who drove back to Miriam's House and met me in my office to explain. It seemed that Latrice had a scheme with one of the employees at Ames. She would shoplift an item and return it another day for a refund, claiming to have lost the receipt. The employee accomplice, stationed behind the complaints desk, would give her the cash. Later, they would split the proceeds. But management had become suspicious and alerted security personnel. That Sunday, they tailed Latrice to the toy department, watched her pick up a doll and walk out of the store. The first thing Faye knew about any of this was when a security guard approached the van and told her to get out.

Grateful they'd believed us, Faye had promised to take no more than three hours to go back to Miriam's House and search Latrice's room for stolen merchandise that she then would return to the store.

We decided Faye would go to Latrice's room, retrieve the contraband, and return it to the defrauded store, only calling me if she needed help. I left her to her task, shaking my head, and went back to my apartment to seek a return to my Sunday quiet mode. But just as I sat down with a cup of tea and my book, the phone rang. The conversation went something like this:

"Carol, I know you don't like to work on Sundays, but I just have to tell you. There's a lot of stuff in here, and some of it's wrapped in Christmas paper. Do you think it's all stolen?"

"Shouldn't we just assume it is? Does it look like Ames stuff?"

"Yeah. Well, the things that aren't wrapped are from Ames. Should I open the wrapped ones?"

By then, I was just too curious to let this go, not to mention Faye had an agreement to take the loot back and I didn't want in any way to renege on this for fear she might yet be arrested. "Sure, open the wrapped ones." While I waited, I imagined Latrice standing in the toy department and taking time to lovingly pick out the perfect gift for her grand baby: "Hmmmm, should I steal the doll or the stuffed bear?" I giggled.

Meanwhile, over the phone, I could hear the sounds of rustling paper. "Wait, this has a tag on it. Oh my God, Carol, it's for you! This tag has your name on it."

"Really? There's a Christmas present for me? Open it! I want to know what she, um . . . got for me."

More rustle of paper. "A bath set. Powder, shower gel, body mist. Lavender."

"I love lavender! How did she know that?" I said, caught up in the excitement and contemplating running down the hall to join the fun, Sunday quiet or no Sunday quiet. "Find yours."

Sounds of packages being lifted and inspected. "Here's one for Elsie, and Donna . . . here's mine!"

Sounds of ripping paper. "A scarf and hat set, goes perfectly with my new winter coat."

"Oh, that's so nice. What's in the rest of the packages? We can tell the others later."

It was larceny, not generosity, a distinction that eluded me in that surreal moment. I listened, glued to the phone and still giggling as Faye opened the packages. We kept a mental list so that we could tell the others what Latrice . . . got for them. We were having far more fun than we should have been, what with the nature of the crime and the fact that Latrice was probably even then languishing in a cell at the fifth district police station.

And we inevitably had to face cold reality and take everyone's gifts, even those we considered ours, back to Ames.

For years afterward, the approach of Christmas always found us in dramatic retelling of The Story of the Christmas Thief, embellished with lamentations about having to return "our" presents. But I did try to make it up to Faye.

That Christmas, I gave her a pair of toy handcuffs. Pink. I had purchased them at Ames.

CHAPTER NINETEEN

Gina really got on my nerves. Perhaps it was because I was still deeply fatigued with lingering effects of Lyme disease when she was admitted in fall of 1999 and lacked patience in general, But before I learned to love most things about her—crooked smile, ever-present bag of Starlight mints, joyous habit of flipping up the volume on the dining-room stereo and sashaying around the tables, her sense of fun—I could not love how she would make almost any circumstance into a complaint, nor the whining tone she employed to do it. She would twit Tim if the van was dusty or if bird droppings marred the hood or wind shield. When I placed the plant-basket hooks to the right of the front door, she complained that they would look better on the left. If I made pancakes for Sunday breakfast, she pouted if they were not blueberry, and if they were, she wished loudly for blueberry syrup to go on them.

I can see her coming down the hall, a middle-aged but young-looking black woman with short-cropped hair outlining her small, shapely skull, expressive eyes above a lopsided grin, pretty face with a flawless complexion. I see her in a well-coordinated outfit, often red, often tight, always in the ineffable Gina style. I see her impromptu performances of characters she'd seen on TV or in movies and the way she seemed to revel in our watching her. Never have I known a woman so needy of attention.

While I was still tired most of the time and short-tempered, Gina was one resident that required more energy than I had to give her. If I needed to learn patience despite fatigue and discomfort, Gina was by far my best teacher.

"It be like a jail up in here. I may as well be back in Lorton."

I was in the kitchen, cleaning up after a Sunday breakfast in early November, but Gina's penetrating tones easily reached me from where she sat in the dining room. I sighed and tried to ignore her, but my resistance was low. I was really tired after the morning on my feet.

Gina had just that week been assigned an early curfew after a misstep involving meeting attendance, so she was moaning with what she believed was good reason. "No better than jail," she said again, louder. Though she had her back to me I heard her clearly, as she meant me to. *Please let her just shut up*, I thought.

She moved closer to the part of the dining room that looked into the kitchen and began a more detailed complaint about how she now had to come in at six o'clock, and how was that going to help her, and she might as well be on lockdown.

Lockdown? Jail? I snapped. "What are you saying? I've given my life for this place, trying to make it a loving home. How can you call it a jail?"

From the look on her face, I could see that my reaction gratified her. Feeling foolish, I went back to my cleaning. *Like a martyr at the stake*, I thought glumly. I had to stop letting her goad me into lashing out.

The leadership course had begun in November 1999, so by early 2000 I was well into the rhythm of it, excited to be challenged and learning. The best part about the course was the coach assigned to each of the students. Mine was Valerie Graff, a woman so wise and honest that I chose to keep her as my executive coach, in which capacity she continued after the course ended and for the next two years. After that, we regularly brought her in for staff and board workshops.

Between Valerie's coaching and the day-long classes every month, I was beginning to see how to resolve the thorny issues I'd been worrying about, like our dysfunctional staff meetings and how my overly active sense of fairness, coupled with a still lingering desire for approval, allowed me to be manipulated by staff. First, however, I had to get honest about my faulty leadership style and the ways I had set the stage for my own difficulties.

I began working toward what the teachers called a "culture change" at Miriam's House, at first exploring my relations with staff. I met with each individually and asked for perceptions of my leadership. Many said they felt shut down when I asked for feedback but then got defensive, that it was annoying when I told them to speak up but then insisted on having the answers and the last word myself, and that my arguments with Faye made them reluctant to confront me. Most of it was stuff I already knew at some level, but that didn't keep it from being hard to hear from them. Yet as I sat there, hugely uncomfortable, I realized I was finally doing what we had been asking the women to do every day for years. We asked them to face honestly the crises, failures, and disastrous relationships caused by their addictions. We asked them to get counseling and be willing to receive feedback and criticism from the counselors and from us. We asked them to confront the behaviors that had brought them down.

And they did. Like Kimberly, sober, living independently, and holding down a part-time job. But it wasn't just success stories. It was Alyssa, who'd got out into the city even when very ill, who'd never given up on her mother. It was Sasha, who had the courage to admit she could not manage her girls. It was Tamara, making friends with me over tofu and chitlins despite my inability to understand her or the way illness sapped her strength and patience. It was Janelle's dignity, Little Karen's sweetness, Muriel's spirit. It was all of them, sitting at their friends' deathbeds and then attending funeral after funeral, handing one another tissues and laying consoling arms over shaking shoulders.

If they could, each in her own way, find the courage to embrace growth and change, then so could I. And more important, I had no right to expect the women to do it if I could or would not do it myself.

After my individual meetings with staff, we created an ad hoc committee that presented a plan for changing the format and procedures at staff meeting. We improved communication between shifts and from day to day. We engaged Valerie in a series of workshops to help us build better relations and improve our teamwork. Though I didn't know it then, this work would evolve naturally into an even more challenging task: a series of workshops on racism and diversity that started in 2005 and didn't end until late in 2009.

Once we took the advice of the ad hoc committee and restructured staff meeting to be deliberately inclusive of every voice and disciplined as to time and topic, I actually began to look forward to those meetings. We were more productive, a better team. Faye and I maintained a truce, somewhat uncomfortably at first, but that formed a foundation for what would become a good working relationship within a few years. And I found out that decisions made through an inclusive process in a group of very different people were often the best ones. It wasn't easy getting used to weighing opposing opinions and relinquishing control, but I sure did like how much better the organization ran.

And, of course, there was Gina. By this time, early 2000, I had developed a deep affection for her. It was tinged with frustration, but I accepted that as part of the reality of knowing Gina.

It seemed we were always taking her to the ER, and we came to believe she harbored a perverse enjoyment of the attention that came with these visits. She developed a particularly annoying habit: she'd wait until eleven o'clock or midnight to decide she was in need of urgent care. It did not matter that we would check on her regularly when her breathing seemed labored, offering to take her to the emergency room or call 911. I even developed a proactive routine designed to get her to the ER at a reasonable hour. It worked well in theory, but when theory met Gina, theory took a dive.

The routine became something of a script.

"Gina, the nurses tell me that you've had trouble breathing this afternoon. I'm on duty tonight and want you to know I'll take you to the ER or call 911." I would look at her hopefully, searching for the Holy Grail of communicating with Gina: a glimmer of cooperation.

"No, I'm okay."

"Really, I'd like to do it now if you're feeling poorly."

"I'm okay."

"Gina," I would go on, a desperation in my voice that I suspected she enjoyed hearing, "I really do not want to get up in the middle of the night again with you in crisis. You can tell if you're going to continue having trouble, so let's just go now if we're headed there anyway."

"I said I'm okay."

She knew and I knew and we both knew that the other knew I was powerless here. If and whenever she said she had to go to the ER, Miriam's House's would ensure she got there. When a PCA called me, of course I would not say to forget it, I'd already offered and she'd told me she was okay.

Finally it occurred to me that she enjoyed these little sessions. I stopped doing them and resigned myself to the late-night crises. One week we were at the Washington Hospital Center ER three nights, including two nights in a row. The staff was able to match our faces with our names that fall. Yet the redeeming feature of these exhausting nights was Gina herself. Her power of observation and penchant for humorous commentary were already becoming legend at Miriam's House.

***

"Uh oh." Gina, sitting next to me in the triage area of Washington Hospital Center emergency room, poked at me with her elbow.

I jumped. "What?"

Gina had been having so much trouble breathing during the ride to the ER from Miriam's House that she'd hung her head out the window, snuffling at the cold night air like a spaniel on an outing. Her exclamation startled me into getting ready to leap out of my chair and demand oxygen for her.

"She's coming." Gina was peering sideways at an elderly woman in a wheelchair about ten feet away from us. Her breathing was still wheezy, but she was distracted for the moment, so I relaxed and tracked her line of vision across the crowded room.

"Hush, Gina. She's not going to hurt you. She's just old and a little odd, maybe. Leave her alone."

"I will if she leave me alone." Her tone was dark, as though she were confronting a grave threat. "I don't trust her." Gina was wheezing between phrases but so intent upon the woman that she seemed not to notice.

I told Gina, a tad impatiently, that the old lady was no threat. Then I looked more closely. The woman seemed disoriented and there was no one attending to her—not unusual in a busy ER—nor was there anyone nearby who looked like family. She exuded scruffiness, with wildly out of control and wispy gray hair, threadbare clothing, and only one shoe. The unshod foot badly needed a podiatrist. I couldn't look at it, so I glanced up at her face.

Her eyes were fixed on Gina. "Oh, I see what you mean. Maybe she recognizes you."

"No." Gina shoved her chair closer to mine. *Wheeze.* "She be creeping me out."

About to reassure her, I stopped short as the woman reached the one shod foot to the floor, placed her heel down, strained, and rolled the chair ever so slightly forward. Toward us. We froze. Again she drew up her foot and put her heel down. The chair advanced another quarter revolution of its wheels. She was making slow, shaky, yet steady progress across that waiting room, unblinking eyes fixed on Gina.

"I told you! She's coming!"

Gina's sudden, fierce whisper pierced my rapt attention and startled me. I jumped and snickered.

"Oh, yeah, real funny." *Wheeze.* "You wouldn't laugh if she was coming for you."

Heartlessly I pointed out how slowly the woman was making progress, and that we'd probably be long gone by the time she made it much closer. Considering that the typical ER visit lasted a minimum of five hours, my calculation might have been off, but it did serve to distract Gina. Her face took on the expression I loved, slightly crooked smile just beginning to form, eyes alight. "Yeah, you right, she ain't gonna get close.

And if she do"—*wheeze*—"you can just sneak around behind her and back her up some." *Wheeze.*

"Well, I don't know about that."

Gina leaned in close, nose to my ear but eyes cut way to the side in order to monitor the progress of our new friend. She imitated the tone of an announcer on an old-time radio science-fiction drama.

"Closer she comes." *Wheeze.* "Step by step." *Wheeze.* The hoarse whisper rose a bit as the woman's heel descended to the floor, pushed against it, and moved the chair toward us. Gina's grin broadened. She squeezed out the short phrases, grimly sotto voce, between asthmatic breaths. She timed them to the moment the woman's heel hit the floor and lifted up again.

"No one is safe."

Wheeze.

"Closer she comes."

Wheeze.

"Step."

Wheeze.

"By."

Wheeze.

"Step."

Wheeze.

Our aged stalker was all of half a foot closer. Gina's gasping had become measured, slower, as though she'd been practicing a remedy developed by a madly creative physician familiar with both asthma and the odd happenings in an emergency room triage area. Put them together and, voila! Breathing therapy.

Focused on her drama, Gina didn't hear the charge nurse call her name. I nudged her. "We're up. We only waited an hour this time."

Throwing one last glance at the woman—who, without missing a beat (*Step. By. Step.*) seemed to have shifted her attention to the person in the chair next to us—Gina got up and followed the nurse to a bay in the treatment area. Immediately demanding a chair for me, she got up on the gurney and sighed.

"Guess we'll never know what she wanted."

We settled in for the long night.

***

One of the worst decisions I ever made at Miriam's House I made in late 1999 when I admitted a family without consulting with or even obtaining basic buy-in from my staff. Once I'd heard their story, I really didn't think much about the admission qualifications of the four boys, ages six to eleven, and their mother. They qualified in the basic ways. Nickie was living with AIDS, they were homeless, the boys were all under thirteen, and we had enough rooms.

What I was ignoring was that years before we'd instituted a policy of limiting families to three children per mother, a practical restriction for our small community. Mothers sometimes needed intensive support and parenting training. Adults and children shared the community spaces, so any parenting or behavior difficulties were magnified by proximity. The resident interns provided most of the respite care we offered with an eagerness and creativity that was touching and helpful, but they couldn't be expected to fill all gaps. And the rest of the staff were not hired to be babysitters or parents. These were all good reasons for limiting the number of children per mother. But once I heard why this family was homeless, I ignored all that.

DC officials called me about Nickie and her boys when they were being housed in a hotel room paid for by the Red Cross. The family qualified for emergency relief after their house had burned during summer 1999. As the flames spread, everyone ran out thinking someone else had picked up the baby girl, the boys' sister. They were huddled, panic-stricken, on the sidewalk when Nickie screamed that her baby was inside. Luke, the youngest boy and only five at the time, raced back into the house to find her. Firefighters found him collapsed indoors, overcome by smoke. They found the baby sister dead in her crib. Luke stayed long months at Children's Hospital fighting for his life while the rest of his family was cared for and provided housing by Red Cross. The family was reunited after Luke was released, but they stayed in the hotel because there was no question of independent housing for this family. Nickie, ill with AIDS and its complications, limited in cognitive ability, and emotionally traumatized by her life and the death of her baby, couldn't work and was living on Aid to Dependent Families. No one believed she could manage without a lot of support. So they called Miriam's House.

It didn't occur to me that I myself had instituted the three-children-per-mother rule. Once I'd heard this harrowing tale and met the two younger boys. I assumed that, like me, other staff members would automatically agree to admit the too-large family. So rather than remember what I'd learned in my leadership course, which was to lay the groundwork with discussions that dealt with objections and anticipated difficulties, I merely told staff they were coming.

All the while, I had to ignore some very strong signals coming from Nickie herself. She spoke vaguely, relying on simple, noncommittal statements to signal agreement or understanding that she probably was not feeling. She moved in a slow, slack-bodied haze of imprecision. Her personal hygiene was atrocious, her clothing looking as though it had been tossed out by a previous owner as too hopelessly stained or ragged for donation. How did I think she could manage four boys?

Angie and I prepared their rooms while I stubbornly pretended the rising discontent among staff was not happening. We purchased toys, games, and better furniture for the rec room on the ground floor. We ensured the continuation of court-ordered family counseling, individual counseling for each, and parenting classes for Nickie. We established a strong connection with the dedicated people at Nickie's church who promised support and respite care. Otherwise, all I thought about was getting the family home with us.

The bedrooms at Miriam's House were connected by pocket doors that could be closed and locked if occupied by individual adults, or opened to make a suite if occupied by a mother and children. We put the two oldest boys, David and Robert, in one suite of two rooms on the first floor and created a three-room suite across the hall for Nickie and the two youngest. The children grinned widely when led into their rooms.

"I get my own room?"

"That bed for me? Just me?"

For the first week or so, life with the new family was fairly peaceful, although the general tension level in the house rose. Some conflict was unavoidable, I told myself. Four young boys, even when they are trying to behave well, bring a certain amount of confusion with them, making a change that rattled some of the women. I monitored the situation during my duty shifts and made regular walks around the building on other evenings, checking in with the intern and PCA and saying hello to Nickie and the boys. For the first week I saw nothing that I wouldn't expect to see in such a situation and so felt hopeful about our ability to help this family. But then, predictably, the children became less wary and more comfortable, and Nickie relaxed into what we soon learned was her usual parenting style of vacant-eyed neglect. The deterioration began, faster, more dramatic, and far more traumatic than ever I could have anticipated.

Each boy, either separately or together, began to exhibit explosive tempers that were all the more shocking because we had experienced their sweet, fun side for several days. Arthur, nine, cursed in a way that appalled even the most hardened of residents and left staff tremendously unsure how to handle him. Any of them could lose control at any time, throwing food or toys or school books, fighting verbally and physically with one another, refusing loudly or profanely to do homework or finish a meal. That meant that we were, especially at mealtime (if you could call it that, their mother seeming to have little concept of nutrition or time) and bedtime, struggling with a furious child or two. Or three. Or four.

The mothers who had lived with us at Miriam's House so far had exhibited a range of parenting skills from exemplary to poor to borderline abusive. The latter we always attended to swiftly, mandating parenting classes and counseling for the mother and counseling for the children, providing respite care and appropriate support at the house, always maintaining close supervision. Nickie had been in counseling and parenting classes since before she arrived. But poor Nickie was as ineffective a parent as we had ever seen. Overwhelmed by her own physical and mental health issues, daily on the move from one doctor appointment to another and then to numerous counseling sessions or classes with the boys, she was also exhausted. If she had parenting skills, she may have been too fatigued to employ them.

The effect was that we were trying to parent the boys in Nickie's stead and at the same time finding ways to encourage and equip her to take over. After a month of this and despite my close supervision and ready presence, most staff members gave up in alarm or anger or both. They argued, justifiably, that this was beyond their abilities and not in their job descriptions. Staff meetings became dreadful again as people voiced fear, anger, and dismay on this one subject that took over our two-hour weekly sessions. I did my best to offer suggestions and bring advice from the counselors, practical measures that, in an atmosphere so rife with emotion, made as little impression as a single drop of oil on water at a rolling boil. Faye was wondering aloud and often why such a large family had been admitted despite our policy of no more than three children per mother, a charge we all knew could be laid at my feet but which I was too overwhelmed to address.

Then Angie's brother died and she took an extended leave, saying she might be back in January.

I threw myself into the task of making it all work, feeling responsible for the mess and having to take over for Angie until we found a new program manager. In my stubborn attention to these children Tim recognized the unresolved baggage I carried about the young boy I'd left when I ended my first marriage back in my twenties. He said so, but I didn't, or couldn't, answer or even reflect on it. I had work to do.

I reached back many years for the knowledge and skills I'd gained while earning a bachelor's degree in elementary education. I personally supervised the kids' bedtimes for several weeks beginning in December and into the New Year, creating a routine with clear limits around book reading and lights out. I instituted a system of points and rewards for the boys' good behavior, cooperation with homework, and mealtime. Tim and I took them on outings to the skating rink and to the Christmas tree on the Mall. Donna and I took them to Chuck E. Cheese's once or twice. On Saturdays, they attended church for most of the day, a break enjoyed by all of us left at the house. I gave up my precious Sunday quiet to help control and entertain the boys with trips to a nearby playground or park, thereby also giving Nickie time to rest. Tim took them out for ice cream a couple of times.

But those outings could turn frightening at any moment, and so we were always on edge with them even when having fun. One otherwise happy trip to the playground ended badly when, on the walk home, Arthur decided he wanted to go to the store for candy. I told him he had to check in with his mother first. He made a break from us, but I grabbed his arm, struggling madly with him on the corner down the street from Miriam's House, feeling ridiculous but desperate to get him home. He shrugged out of the coat and I was left holding it, watching him run away. The other three boys were already wandering into the street, so I angrily threw the coat down, shouted after him to pick it up on his way back, and went to gather his brothers. We got to the house and I rushed in to find Nickie. As the boys took off their coats, Nickie and I sped out the front door to find Arthur. There he was, just up at the corner and on his way home, pockets full of candy and carrying his coat.

I began to dread reading the daily logbook notes written the night before by a helplessly disheartened intern, with their tales of violent anger, and bedtimes and mealtimes ignored. I felt gratitude for Jan, who would comfort and pray with the resident who lived below Nickie's three-room suite when she complained of being unable to sleep for all the noise. After a while, Desaray, a resident intern who had begun working with us just a couple of months before the family moved in, learned to see the sweeter aspects of the boys' personalities, and tried out her own gentle support and encouragement of them. But that was well into January, and until then, Donna—the only person who could get the boys to listen—and I were the ones who fought to make it all work. I relied completely on her staunch support.

By late January it finally began to look as though our methods were having a positive effect. The boys' behavior slowly changed. Meals, homework, and bedtimes were quieter, less fraught with frustration. We even began to have fun with them. Desaray reported congenial games of Sorry! after helping the boys with their homework. Jan found a couple of books that made getting to bed more pleasant. And Nickie did a better job keeping her own room clean and getting her sons to clean theirs. She began to cook more often and made her first tentative forays into practicing the parenting skills she was learning.

From where this hurting and damaged family found the courage to begin trusting us enough to allow their softer and more vulnerable sides to emerge, I could not tell, but I admired them for it. And I felt relieved. I was able to relax on evenings and weekends I wasn't on duty, no longer on tenterhooks that I might be called downstairs to restrain a wild boy or problem-solve with a wretched intern. There were still difficult times, but we saw Nickie's attempts to discipline and nurture her brood. Staff members became more willing to attempt a relationship with them. I noted with awe the bare beginnings of transformation on the part of these children who had been entrusted to our care and who seemed to be beginning to believe in it.

The change was short-lived.

Faye called me on a Sunday afternoon in early February, speaking agitatedly and incoherently about a knife found in the dining room and David screaming, "She gonna kill me!"

I raced downstairs.

David, sullen and guarded, would give me little information. We later speculated that he was trying to protect his mother. But Faye had found a knife under her coat in the dining room just after David screamed. Several residents reported they saw Nickie chasing after him with the knife in her hand. Faye and I did our best to settle the community, now in an uproar, and ensure David's safety for the night by locking his door and taking the key away from Nickie. The PCA on overnight shift checked on him every half hour. The next day, Monday, we called Child Protective Services. Specialists interviewed the boys, took them from school that very day, and placed them in the foster-care program. And, with a sea change that took fewer than six hours, our house became very quiet indeed.

Nickie stayed with us while she looked for an apartment. Bitterness and hurt made her uncooperative, so she talked to none of us and joined no community activity. When she could get away with it, she ate take-out food in her room, despite our pleas about bugs and the mess. We drove her to supervised meetings with the boys and supported her presence in counseling and parenting classes. We tried to connect with her, but in her eyes we had taken her family, and there was no prospect of reconciliation. We all felt it, too, but especially me, the architect of the whole ungodly mess.

In late spring of 2000, Nickie found an apartment she could afford. Her case manager and Yvonne—the LPN we'd hired to supplement the work of the RN—and I had rejected one or two earlier choices as being unsanitary or otherwise unsuitable. This was better, but still poorly kept and surely roach-ridden. Nickie didn't care. She wanted out of Miriam's House. On the Saturday after her court-appointed lawyer approved the move, we hauled her bags and boxes out of our house. I drove the car, and Tim drove the van to the apartment in Northeast DC. The car had a flat tire on the way, but I barely minded the long wait in the cold, dank, oily-smelling garage. While Tim took Nickie, the van, and its contents over to the apartment, and I waited for the tire to be changed, within me relief that it all was over contended with some small, not named, and fracturing place that expected no comfort.

***

After Nickie left, I realized I'd been grinding away at work without respite. Even after the boys had gone, her very presence in the house had been a reminder of the disturbing and ultimately terrifying saga of their time with us. During the spring of 2000 I made myself look around to see what was going well.

Kimberly often dropped by to hang out, have a meal, and show us how well she was doing. She had maintained her sobriety, stayed at Shalom House, and even obtained a part-time job cleaning clinic offices in the evenings. She'd gained enough weight to make her arms and legs looked less like stork appendages. Her demeanor was more of confidence and joy than it used to be. We were pleased, and clearly so was she. In our world, where success might be measured by getting dressed without help or making it to three NA/AA meetings a week, seeing a former resident doing well, working a job, and living in greater independence meant so much. We made joyful notes in the daily logbook whenever we saw her and encouraged her return visits.

Our newest staff member was Yvonne, an LPN. She was both a helpful colleague and one of the few willing to speak the truth to me. She had a great sense of humor, much like mine, and we got along well.

Faye and I, our briefly revived antagonism resolved once the boys were gone, were forced to get along after Angie resigned. Faye stepped into the breach, meeting with me every Sunday and spending hours on the phone during the week discussing the residents and their issues, helping me so willingly and with such insight that, although the extra work stretched me in some ways to my limit, I never felt unequal to it. This was, as it had been from the beginning, where Faye and I became allies: in our love for and support of the women of Miriam's House.

As if the fates had turned a benign eye upon our work, either as reward for us getting along or in sympathy for all we'd been through, we entered again into a season of relative calm. There began what I think of now as a unique time at Miriam's House, a time of women large of personality and vivid of speech, entertaining seekers of attention, women whose quirks and oddities were admired almost as much by the rest of us as by they themselves.

My coaching with Valerie—a coach so relentlessly challenging I'd say to her, "I'm *paying* you to do this to me?"—was beginning to bear fruit. I noticed it mostly in how much more comfortable I had become with staff. I grew to rely on Yvonne's honesty and loyalty, Faye's willingness to give so much of herself to our work, Donna's rock-steadiness in a crisis, Elsie's ability to overcome initial reluctance toward change and invest in it. I felt more compassion for the low self-esteem burdening many of the PCAs and worked out ways, like a PCA Appreciation Tea one spring afternoon, to help bolster their confidence.

As I backed off my need to have all the answers, Yvonne spoke up more and was taking on a respected role among staff. As I delegated decisions and tasks to individuals and small groups, not only did they become more invested, but I had more time for myself and was less fatigued. The change spilled over to my work with the residents. I could just enjoy Gina and her theatrics, bear with equanimity her constant whining. I could hang out in the dining room or watch TV with them without feeling self-conscious and different. Responsibility weighed on me less heavily. I was beginning to feel competent, equal to the monumental task I'd set for myself with barely an inkling of what it would take.

Perhaps I could, after all, stay.

CHAPTER TWENTY

Miriam's House, especially with Gina in residence and Kimberly visiting, was a lively and amusing place. Add Terri, and we had quite a theater.

Terri, who moved in during July of 2000, matched Gina in humor and will to entertain, though not, thankfully, in her desperate need for attention. To look at Terri was to know that she was a person of wit. Her long, narrow face with its slightly protruding eyes and humorous mouth would assume expressions of the gravest sincerity while telling the most egregious lies, the movement of her skinny arms adding emphasis to everything she said, be it truth or dare, fiction or nonfiction. Short in stature, slight in body, oversize in personality, Terri possessed a charm that, similar to Kimberly, made it impossible to stay angry or upset with her. And with Terri in the house, even a nighttime power outage could be fun.

Miriam's House was situated a block away from construction of a new Metro line, meaning we underwent regular power outages. Most of these occurred at night. Tim and I would get up to perform backup routines for the security and phone systems, and then Tim would go back to bed. I would stay up to be with the women who came downstairs.

These were women untrusting of the night. Aroused by the sudden dark and quiet, they would emerge sleepy-eyed from their rooms. So we came together, like moths seeking the dim glow of the emergency lights, bathrobes fluttering about our ankles, slippered feet shuffling, gathering in the front hallway or dining room to speak in hushed tones and listen to the unaccustomed dark's unnerving quiet, taking assurance from one another's presence.

**

On the night of Terri's first power outage she was not with us as we settled into the dining room, faces awash in the pale yellow glow of emergency bulbs. For some reason the traffic light on the intersection just outside the dining-room windows was working. From the corner of my eye I noticed the changing colors—red, then green, then yellow; red, then green, then yellow. We were quiet.

Well, most of us were.

"Shit, man, where the hell did everybody go? Why you all down here and ain't told me? I hate these damn blackouts. Can't sleep in the dark."

We couldn't yet see her, but we knew who was coming. The kitchen door opened. Out of the shadows and into our quiet emerged Terri's tiny figure, clad in a midthigh-length white T-shirt and her skinny legs ludicrously stuck into oversize hiking shoes, laces flapping. She flickered a flashlight around the dining room as she came in. This was Terri in a state of preparedness.

We perked up.

"Hey, Terri."

"Whatcha doing in them clothes?"

"What the hell you got them boots on for? Ain't no flood."

"You late, girl, we been here ten minutes."

"Stop shining that damn light in my eyes."

"Let's tell stories," she said and flopped into a chair. With no pause for a response, Terri launched into the tale of the kidnapping that happened just before she moved in. Gesticulating, eyes shining in the dim light, she swore never to do nothing like that again. "I shouldn't never of gone there, Georgia Avenue be one of them trigger places for me. All them addicts and dealers and I know most of 'em. Plus I shouldn't never of got in that car, but you know what you do when you be jonesing for a hit."

Nods all around.

There was another person in the car, a nice-looking young woman, and so Terri had thought it would be okay to get in. The driver told her he had to get to the place where the drugs were, you know, had to find the drug man. "But then he drive all the way out to I-don't-know-where, way the hell out in Maryland land and I get scared. And so I start begging the guy cuz I don't know where the hell we at, but he ain't looking at me or even acting like he notice."

Was it getting darker? I glanced up at the emergency light to see if it had dimmed. Terri saw me. She paused. We waited.

"Well, I ain't know where I was. And then I could see the other girl, the one I thought was okay, she was scared, too, and she ain't acting like she know the guy. She say to him to please let us out. That make me real scared."

Red, then green, then yellow. Red, then green, then yellow.

Terri told the guy she had AIDS and needed her medication and would get terribly sick if she didn't get it and please *please* let her out and all the while crying. The other passenger began to holler at him, and Terri was begging, begging, and the other woman said, take me, take me, but let the sick girl go.

Silence.

Terri finished in a rush. "Must have been too much confusion for him so he lets me out, side of the road. Left me there. Didn't know where the hell I was at."

Terri looked down at her boots and shuddered, or was it just the rippling weight of light on her slight, white-clad form? She wondered if the other one made it.

We didn't ask how Terri got back. We just knew she did, because here she was.

"It be scary as hell out there, man." Terri glanced around. We nodded. Tiny and frail, she seemed impossibly delicate sitting there in our dining room. I thought I heard her whisper "Hope she made it."

Red, then green . . .

"Scary as shit out there!" We jerked in surprise as Terri rose up to stamp around the room's perimeter in that ridiculous footwear. "Scary as *shit.*"

Enough of the late-night confessions, Terri was ready to be outrageous. She circled the room then sat again in her chair, raised her leg and clomped an oversize boot onto the table.

"Girl, you trifling!"

"Get that big old ugly thing off our table."

"We gotta eat up in here."

Terri grinned while the others united to shove the boot off the table. She jumped up again.

"We need some music. Time to dance."

***

Terri's humor, Kimberly's happy visits, and Gina's antics provided needed relief during the summer of 2000 when I found myself drawn into a fight not of my choosing, but unavoidable. The leader of an organization serving women, many of them our residents, had once before made public complaints about Miriam's House and me, when Sasha, whom she knew and loved, had died. She began again that summer, using one of our women, Hattie, as a means to attack us. Though we never knew the woman's true motivation, Faye figured it had something to do with her being a person of color and me, white.

Hattie had a twelve-year-old daughter, Keisha. They'd been with us for a few months when Hattie flung herself into open rebellion. She refused to honor visitor rules, stayed out past curfew, and finally, disappeared for three extra days after a permitted weekend away. To a certain extent, we knew she was following the instructions of the other executive director, who told Hattie she didn't have to obey our rules. We found out that the she had also anonymously listened in on a phone conversation between Hattie and me, then composed a letter using my words against me, an unprofessional and unethical act that fueled our anger and made work with Hattie even more difficult.

But it became really bad when Hattie began using her daughter as a means to flaunt her independence. Our policy for mothers stated they must always be in direct supervision of their children unless they'd previously arranged with us for respite care. But Hattie refused to be home for Keisha's return from school at 3:30 p.m., leaving the child without direct supervision. After several weeks of fruitless repetition of the rules, levying of consequences that had no effect, and numerous warnings that we would have to ask Keisha to remain outside until Hattie got home, we one day refused Keisha entrance into the house. The weather was warm and sunny, and the PCA, Donna, and I checked obsessively to make sure Keisha was all right out there on the patio throughout the thirty minutes until Hattie returned. But for long afterward I felt extremely uncomfortable about that decision. And for long afterward, Keisha would not speak to me. Even their eventual move out to an apartment, which should have been a relief, only made me feel worse.

In November 2000 we hired a new PCA. Linda was slender and energetic, a woman with a flair for fashion, a wonderful rapport with the women, and a way of making the place homey. If the dining-room tables were decorated with bud vases, I knew Linda had been at the rose bushes. When we held a special event, Linda would be the one in the red-velvet pants suit spangled with gold, red shoes on her feet, and a gold beret on her head. Beloved of staff and residents, Linda's never-failing good humor even suffered without complaint our open amusement at how her narcoleptic tendencies had her nodding off during staff meeting and then starting awake to a mumbling continuation of whatever we'd been talking about when she'd fallen asleep. She could even drop off at the dining-room table, sandwich in hand, slumped ever so slightly over her plate. After we spoke to her about that, Linda wouldn't trust herself to sit down during her shift. Except for her breaks, she kept upright and moving for the duration. And though she continued to fall asleep in meetings, and the interns sometimes mentioned that Linda nodded off in the van on the way to do the week's grocery shopping, we said nothing. As long as she wasn't the one driving, we felt she was entitled to a little rest.

***

Early in our time at Miriam's House, we'd developed the habit of framing photos of house life and hanging them on the hallway wall outside the kitchen. Photos taken during renovation, others of cookouts on the patio, children and Tim playing in the living room, holiday and anniversary parties, women dancing in the dining room, some residents and me goofing around, and PCAs in the kitchen: the wall became a chronicle of our years together. My favorites were the ones of women who had died. Of those, I especially cherished one that commemorated our only Christmas with Crystal, who was with us for just six months. That photo is paired in my mind with a memory of Easter 2001. In the Christmas photo she and I are standing together at the tree, deciding where to place an ornament, and we're smiling. In the Easter memory I'm holding her candy-and-gift-filled basket, and I am alone.

***

"Where should I put this one? This Santa Claus with the funny face?" I put it in her hand, which closed around it, thoughtfully hefting its weight and measuring the length of the tasseled hat.

She said it needed a big spot and tipped her head to one side. We'd been working on that tree for a while, and even though the only tree-decorating scheme to which Miriam's House could lay claim was to load it with as much bling as possible, there was always someone pointing out bare spots.

I mentioned a spot between a red ball and a straw angel.

"No," she said, "Santas do not go next to angels."

In the photo we're looking at the tree, she a bit in front of me and in full profile. A glimpse of red ribbon, matching the red number-twenty-one football jersey she wears, holds tiny corkscrews of hair in place. A silver earring gleams in her left ear. She's touching the tree and smiling.

"Okay," I said, "here's a little green stocking next to a big space with a teddy bear on the other side."

"Good."

The photo shows me hanging the ornament with Crystal beside me, serenely smiling. I am the one to actually place that funny-faced Santa because Crystal couldn't see to place it herself. She was blind as a result of an opportunistic infection that had invaded her brain a year before.

She turned her head and called out, "Any more bare spots?" She hoped, I guessed, to get Gina's opinion. Gina, who would have placed decorations three deep on that tree until it was as cluttered as her room.

"Gina went to get some snacks," I said peering into the dining room, "and it looks like all the food is out. You hungry?"

In response, Crystal grabbed my arm. We navigated carefully through the boxes emptied of their holiday decorations and the paper, bags, and discarded ornaments scattered on the floor. We stopped at the snack table in the dining room, where she asked if I'd put out the popcorn and chocolate yet.

My mother was still making a gift of a five-pound box of chocolates and a large, decorated can full of three flavors of popcorn for our holiday celebrations. She'd have it waiting for Tim and me at Thanksgiving, when we visited family in Delaware. The residents counted on the tradition of Mom's treats, and even Crystal, celebrating her first Christmas with us, knew about it.

Crystal wanted to know what else was on the table. I listed a cheese-and-cracker-and-veggie tray. Chips. And dips, nacho cheese and french onion. Some fruit. Cookies and brownies. To drink, the usual: water, fruit juices, Coke, Diet Coke, ginger ale, diet Sprite. As I went through the list, Crystal stood quietly, listening. I asked her what she wanted. She said her boys would get there soon, so she'd better fix their plates. Crystal had been at Miriam's House long enough to experience how quickly food disappeared. I put out three of the paper Santa Claus plates, one for each of her sons and one for her, and piled them according to her instructions: "Joey likes the caramel corn, and put some nacho dip on there, with potato chips, that's his favorite. Jeremy likes the cheese corn, lots, and you better put some carrots on there, too, for both of 'em, and each one gets two chocolates." She wanted some fruit, cheese, and crackers.

She smiled as we settled ourselves and the plates at a table to wait for her beloved boys to arrive. Crystal couldn't see it, but the tables were covered with red, green, gold, and blue cloths printed with poinsettias, wreaths, snow scenes, and snowmen. She couldn't see the fake snow sprayed on the windows, or the live poinsettia plants scattered around, or the tiny white twinkle lights strung on the palm tree. She couldn't see that Tim had set fuzzy reindeer antlers on his head, or that I wore my Christmas scarf, that Gloria sported a Santa hat on which red lights blinked, and Cassie, the resident intern that year, had draped a loop of shimmery red garland around her neck.

But she sat there at the table she could not see, with the plates she was not able to prepare for the sons she could not mother, and Crystal smiled. That's why I love the Christmas photo. In it Crystal smiles, an expression that became increasingly rare as the next four months wore on, her health worsened, and her psychosis increased.

***

In January, Crystal began to fear bedtime, delaying our departure by asking for another story or a glass of water. Once or twice she asked me to sing her to sleep. She became fearful whenever a staff member was not within hearing range and would panic until someone could get to her. This made weekends and evenings, when the number of available staff was reduced, rather tricky. Eventually she resolved her fear by following the intern on duty around "like a puppy," one of them reported affectionately.

Her psychiatrist prescribed Haldol, an antipsychotic, to control her agitation and psychosis. The drug did calm her enough so that she could respond to instructions or encouragement given in a quiet, firm tone. But the side effects of this medication made her stagger as though she had no control over her own muscles, bad enough for someone who could see, but disastrous for Crystal, who would get too impatient to wait for help and go careening down hallways and caroming off walls like a cue ball.

Crystal was in the hospital for her February birthday. Donna, Kimberly, another resident, and I took her a cake, but she cried so much over it we left so she could calm down.

Spring 2001 was already an upsetting time, mainly because we were struggling with Terri. She, like Crystal, was in and out of the hospital every few weeks, but she began calling friends to take her to the ER rather than notifying staff. Suddenly we'd have a call from Terri telling us she was admitted to one of the city's hospitals. We would scramble around putting the paperwork together and rush an intern over to get the list of current medications and notification instructions to nurses in charge. And she never wanted us to visit, keeping us in the dark about her health and making us suspicious about what was actually going on. Several suspected that her drinking buddies were slipping booze to her, meaning there may have been bottles around that she would not have wanted us to see.

Among the other residents, random difficulties popped up without respite. Juanita relapsed in March and disappeared for a week. When she returned she showed me large, dark bruises on her back, the result of having been beaten by her drug man. I exclaimed over them in horror, but she shrugged and said, in a matter-of-fact tone, that he had a right to do it because she'd never paid him for the heroin. Two residents, mutually antagonistic, held shouting and cursing matches in the dining room.

We had so many women in the various hospitals that I brought out a chart I'd created in our first year, on which we could keep track of visits and make sure no resident was inadvertently forgotten. Two residents suffered deeply from depression. We worked to connect them with counseling, trying to coax them out of their isolation by extending special invitations to leave their rooms and join the bingo game on Wednesdays or come downstairs for a sobriety anniversary party in the dining room. I attended two poetry slams in which Keisha performed, one at the Borders bookstore on Nineteenth Street and one at her junior high school. Keisha still would not look at or speak to me when I remained late to congratulate her and check in with Hattie.

A particular friend of Crystal's, an older resident who used to sit at a dining-room window and tell her what was going on outside, fell in the bathroom and broke her hip. After twenty days on a ward in Howard Hospital, she died of pneumonia. Crystal, distraught over her friend's death, tumbled into depression. She voiced increasingly desperate complaints about her blindness, so we looked around for therapeutic activities. We bought her a tape recorder and books on tape, which calmed her and alleviated her boredom during the day. But she still wanted her personal bedtime reading to continue.

On a Saturday in late March, Crystal fell in the kitchen while trying to get juice for her boys, who were visiting for the day. She couldn't get up, nor could they help her up. They ran for staff, who helped Crystal to her feet after checking that she was uninjured. The three of them were so upset we called the boys' guardian to come get them and took Crystal to rest in her room. After that, newly insecure, she couldn't or wouldn't manage her sons on their visits. They weren't badly behaved children, but two young boys have a lot of energy and require close supervision. We arranged for another adult to be present during their visits, supplementing or outright taking over the children's care.

I don't remember what illness took Crystal to the ER, but she was admitted into Howard Hospital about ten days before Easter. As usual, we visited her, relaying messages back and forth and bringing items she needed—a comb, her tape recorder, some lotion. Her spirits, already low, plummeted at the news she would not be discharged in time to have Easter at Miriam's House.

I wasn't on duty that Easter weekend except to cook Sunday breakfast. I had thought about checking in with Cassie, the intern on duty, or at least scanning the daily log notes as I usually did. *But I'm too tired,* I told myself, *and it's been a difficult few months. I'd better get some real rest if I want to make it to summer.* I never checked in. On Sunday morning I was too busy distributing Easter baskets and making breakfast to read Cassie's notes from the day before. And so, after I'd finished cleaning up from breakfast, I simply picked up Crystal's Easter basket filled with treats and small gifts and the orange cream rolls she loved so much, and left for the hospital.

She didn't make her usual eager response to my knock on her room door, so I poked my head in. The bed was made with clean sheets pulled tight and smooth. No Crystal. I backtracked down the hall to the nurses' station, assuming she had been transferred to a different room or taken elsewhere for tests.

The station was adorned for Easter in a way that made me imagine some energetic kindergartener had been turned loose with too many decorations and too little supervision. The bulletin board was a chaos of yellow, white, and cute for which the only sign of an interest in neatness was that it kept to the perimeter. I caught the eye of a nurse behind the counter.

"I'm here to visit Crystal in room S412. She's not there, and . . ." I stopped because the woman behind the counter was staring at me, mouth open.

Puzzled, but focused on bringing Easter to Crystal, I explained. "Crystal Myers, I'm talking about. She's been here for at least a week, but she's not in her room just now. Is she getting tests? Or was she moved?" I placed the Easter basket on the counter as though presenting Exhibit A to a judge who, on the very fact of its fragrant and festive presence, would grant me reprieve from the fear already forming in the pit of my stomach.

Lord, why didn't she say something?

The mad kindergartner had tacked cute, yellow, smiling chicks and cute, white, lop-eared bunnies onto the bulletin board behind the speechless, motionless woman. One of the chicks had swiveled on its tack so that its little orange beak was gaping upward and its little clawed feet were grasping pathetically at air. The woman blinked, but said nothing. I babbled. "I just want to see her and give her this basket. I made her favorite rolls this morning. She's not in her room. Where is she?"

I put my hands around the base of the basket, feeling the prickly touch of green plastic grass poking through the weave. "This is her basket. I brought it for her. It's *Easter*."

I felt a choking urge to tell the clearly incompetent woman to move her stationary butt and set that little chick—the one dangling sideways on its tack, the one suddenly irritating the hell out of me—aright.

Another nurse approached the counter, focused her gaze on Crystal's basket, and spoke. "I'm so sorry. Miss Myers died early this morning."

I did not ask what killed her or why we had not been called per the instructions on the contact form that I *knew* we'd made sure was placed in her file and that was *surely* right there at the nurses' station. I picked up the basket with deliberate and delicate care, as though preserving it in perfect condition could make it okay that Crystal would never receive it. The basket and I backed away from the silent nurses and their devastating information. Behind them the chick gawped dementedly.

Back at Miriam's House, relieved no one was on the front patio to see me return still gripping the basket, I slipped through the front door and up the stairs to my office. I sat numbly in my chair for several minutes. She had died. Alone. I could barely think about it. But I had to let people know, so I called Faye and asked her to see me in my office. She stopped short when she saw the look on my face and the basket in my lap.

"Oh no. Oh no, don't tell me. Don't tell me." Faye backed away from me as I had from the nurses, as though introducing a degree of physical distance might somehow turn to good the bad news surely coming.

"I went to give Crystal her Easter basket. She wasn't in her room. They told me she died this morning."

Faye sat down. I repeated what I knew, avoiding any mention of Crystal dying in the dark. We shared the box of tissues. Once we were calmer, Faye left to find the women and announce an emergency meeting in the dining room. I got Crystal's file and called her family, a task I always dreaded but that felt particularly awful this time. Another thought to hold at bay: those newly orphaned boys.

I joined Faye and the women in the dining room. Most of the residents were home from church, so the room was full. They knew we had bad news. They read our faces.

"Didn't know she was that sick. Wish I'd gone to visit yesterday."

"God brought her home, she done suffered too much already."

"On Easter? She died on Easter?"

"She in a better place."

"Do other staff know yet? How you gonna tell them?"

"Oh no, the boys. The boys. What about the boys?"

"Can we have one of them memorial services? After dinner?"

"No, before, before dinner. Sooner. Can we do it sooner?"

We agreed to hold the memorial service in an hour. We set up the living room, putting a photo of Crystal and her boys, the white pillar candle, and the tea lights on the coffee table. We circled the chairs. Someone chose a gospel piece to play. I put my old Bible on the table. Each one who felt she could bear it, came. The rest stayed away.

After the service, after dinner, after making phone calls to staff, I finally had time to read Cassie's daily log notes for the weekend. She had carefully noted, after both her Friday evening and Saturday afternoon visits, that Crystal seemed very ill, shockingly so, given her condition during the preceding week. Horrified, I realized that had I followed my impulse to check in with Cassie, I would have known to go to Crystal on Saturday. But I hadn't, and so Crystal had died by herself in the hospital.

Crystal. Blind. Frightened of the dark. Afraid of being alone.

I had failed her. Broken my promise. And nothing, *nothing* to be done to make it right. Nothing. Nothing.

After a long and frozen while, there surfaced the only thought to hold any consolation at all: *At least I'm here. And there's nowhere else I want to be.*

CHAPTER TWENTY-ONE

The center of community life was the dining room in which, over kitchen noises of clattering pots and frying foods, we danced, sulked, partied, played games, shared meals, fought, broke up fights, memorialized dead friends, and sang with the gospel and oldies stations. That dining room saw a lot of life. For Gina, the dining room also functioned as a stage. Her habit was to turn up the stereo volume upon entering the room, and dance. Others could join her if they chose. Gina liked to dance and she liked attention. But the coup de grace, the performance to end all performances, came courtesy of Sha-nay-nay. The first time I saw Sha-nay-nay (I don't know how to spell it, so this is a phonetic version) was one evening when we were having dinner.

In the middle of a conversation with another resident about a word-search puzzle, I looked up to see a fantastic vision in the doorway.

The face was adorned with Gina's familiar crooked grin but bedaubed with scarlet lipstick and competing for attention with the blond wig perched above it. She wore a red dress. A

tight red dress. And heels. Tall spike heels. After a disdain-
ful glance that swept a crowd struck dumb, this spectacle in
red and blond launched herself into the dining room from the
hand-on-hip pose she'd assumed in the doorway.

I leaped from my chair thinking I'd catch Gi . . . Sha-nay-
nay, who wasn't managing the heels well. But she seemed
unbothered that her otherwise dramatic entrance had been
marred by the failure of a spike-heeled shoe to negotiate the
door sill, catapulting her into the dining room as though from
a slingshot. Noting her composure, I sat back down to watch.

Gina's trademark grin fought with Sha-nay-nay's expression of lofty scorn as she strutted through the dining room,
weaving her precarious way between tables and grabbing onto
the backs of chairs when one or the other ankle proved unequal
to the task of controlling those heels. Terri said something I
couldn't quite catch above the laughter, causing Sha-nay-nay
to stop abruptly. With a withering look, she made with her free
arm a sweeping gesture that ended in a snap of her fingers just
short of Terri's nose.

"Oh no you didn't, girl. Oh no you did not." She weaved her
long neck with that in-out-around sinuous motion that only a
black woman can pull off. She had Attitude.

Our meals grew cold on our plates as we watched. Sha-
nay-nay, after more antics, would clearly have liked to stay longer but, alas, those shoes were her undoing, and she was forced
to retreat. We were left behind, laughing.

***

So enamored were we of the entertainment that we began
regularly demanding Sha-nay-nay, who proved to be as
capricious as Gina herself, emerging only when good and

ready. Or, more likely, when Gina was feeling particularly left out.

If Gina's time at Miriam's House was marked by dramatic ER visits, impromptu dance fests, and the occasional appearance of Sha-nay-nay, Terri's time with us was marked with relapses vehemently denied and readmissions accompanied by vociferous contrition that fooled no one. Terri and Gina were larger than life one at a time, a world unto themselves when at the house together. I suppose it was inevitable that their stories eventually intertwined in a way that accommodated Gina's desire for attention and Terri's addiction.

Terri held the record for relapsing, leaving, staying out for a while, and returning, a pattern she'd established within six months of her admission. Terri actually enjoyed life when she was drinking. She never seemed to get to that "sick and tired of being sick and tired" place that many addicts in recovery say is the reason they turned around. Whenever Terri wanted to come back to Miriam's House it was because she was too ill to continue living the lifestyle of the street. Usually she was referred back to us by a hospital social worker whom she'd told that she was a resident at Miriam's House.

The irony was that Terri would become healthier during her stays with us, just enough so that her renewed strength would grant her the energy to go back out again. And though she would eventually return contrite, swearing she was committed to being sober, Terri never really was sober, the intervals between relapses being too short to be called sobriety. Here was a woman that relapsed five times in six months during her first stay at Miriam's House. In a program that required off-site three- or six-month recovery and treatment after a third relapse, this was unprecedented. Yet we discovered early on that Terri was too ill for most treatment programs, which could be rigorous even for a healthy person. Not to mention that the word *cooperative* was only wishfully—never accurately, though always lovingly—applied to Terri, healthy or sick.

During her first summer with us, Terri relapsed for the fourth time in as many months. We placed her in a three-month drug treatment program that was one of the few willing to admit persons with AIDS. We never learned whether it was due to her illness or her lack of cooperation, but before long she was dropped off at Howard Hospital ER and left there. She called Miriam's House and told the PCA on shift where she was. I was on overnight call, so the PCA contacted me, and I got myself up, dressed, and over to Howard.

It was our habit to accompany our women to the ER unless they expressly wished to be alone. Experience had taught us that they seemed repeatedly to be the last to receive attention. Was it because they were poor, low on the privilege scale, on Medicaid and disabled? Or because they themselves, having learned to grab quickly and even violently for what little attention and care they could get, sometimes alienated the very people trying to help them? By then, I had stopped trying to answer these questions. We just ensured that they had an advocate with them at the ER.

Terri and I together and in an ER bay. These visits, amusing and even fun, run together in my memory, though the pattern is unforgettable.

***

When I arrived, she looked tired. However, Terri tired was not Terri silent.

"Miss Carol, they ain't knowed what to do with me, just wanted to believe I got sick. Didn't even call my doctor, just brought me over here. Fine with me. I'm glad for the rest. You wouldn't believe that program, sitting in them hard-ass chairs forever, then a long walk and more damn meetings. Food was lousy, too. How'm I supposed to get better eating shit like that?"

Terri, for such a small person, had a big voice, but if I had to be at the ER at two o'clock in the morning, I may as well enjoy her. For the entertainment value, maybe, but mostly because I admired her spirit and was loathe to shut her down.

"Man, them counselors was weird. Plonked a dunce cap on my head and sat me on a stool in the hall. A dunce cap, you know, that pointy tall hat, and way too big for me, falling all over my eyes and shit, couldn't see nothing and my neck got tired trying to hold the damn thing up."

"That sounds harsh." I'd heard many stories about the methods some treatment programs used to enforce rules, like women forced to scrub the floor with a toothbrush or wear a sign labeling some "character defect" identified by staff, and although I tried to be professional and simply hint about my aversion to these practices, the fact was that Miriam's House never, ever treated a woman that way.

"They said I was disruptive in groups, but I was just saying my mind. Got no sense of humor over there."

A nurse came in. "The doctor will be in to see you in a few minutes."

"You done said that six hours ago."

"Well, hardly," I murmured, reluctant to interfere but knowing she hadn't been there that long. Yet.

The nurse ignored us both. "Put this under your tongue."

"I be going blind. Can't see nothing." Now she sounded peevish.

"Well, I can see you're looking at it." The nurse waved the thermometer a bit as if to prove her point. Terri, I was sure, scoffed inwardly at this transparent ploy. She squinted, let her gaze go unfocused, and swiveled her head like a bobblehead doll on the dashboard of a pimped-out Cadillac.

"Can't see nothing," she said vaguely.

The nurse gave up and helped Terri, who looked satisfied. Terri had a way of quelling all opposition.

After the nurse left, I was asked to stand at the curtain that divided our bay from the rest of the ER and tell Terri what was going on. Sometimes I opened the curtain a bit so she could watch, too. We hung out for a while, if being at an ER and commenting on the goings-on ("That guy on the stretcher there, ain't that blood I see? He been shot? Go ask."), and deflecting the more outrageous requests ("Are you crazy? I'm not going to walk up to a man lying in bloody sheets on a stretcher and ask him how he got here.") could be called hanging out. The thing was that ER visits with Terri, though they lasted the usual five to seven hours, flew by. I was just along for the ride.

**

I finally left at about five o'clock that morning, after the doctor ordered some tests to help her decide if she would admit Terri. In the end she was not admitted, but when we called the treatment program to retrieve her, they refused. Having dropped her off the night before, they'd apparently washed their hands of her. Although we wanted to make a point of this blatant lack of professionalism, we had no time. The hospital was ready to release her to the street, unacceptable to us because Terri was too ill to be on the street. We were justifiably worried she would use when she was out there. We picked her up from the ER and brought her back to Miriam's House.

Terri continued to relapse at semiregular intervals. As she did, we ran out of treatment programs that either she hadn't yet attended and thoroughly alienated, or that accepted women with AIDS. We had a problem. Our program encouraged long-term commitment from the women, pointedly saying that we would not and could not allow a swinging-door policy, with residents moving in and out at whim. It all came to a head one winter day, with staff members split and defending opposing points of view: we had no choice but to let Terri come back; we could not possibly let Terri come back.

That was one long and contentious staff meeting. At the start, Yvonne informed us that the hospital at which Terri had ended up was ready to discharge her as early as that afternoon. We had to make a decision then and there. Allow her to return, or not?

I had developed some skills recently but was still learning how to mediate conflict in staff meeting. And what made these discussions even harder was that they often drew racial lines between us. White staff tended to advocate for leniency, black staff for strictness.

"She's going to get all the other women using. This is supposed to be a clean and sober house. What are we saying about our rules if she can just keep coming back no matter how often she uses?"

"She comes back in here and they all know she been using. She stinks of it. You don't know what it's like out there, and it's dangerous for everyone when she brings the smell of it in here."

Meaning, I knew, you white people don't know what it's like out there. I couldn't argue with this or that our sobriety policies were of tantamount importance. How could I know what street life was like? All I knew were the stories the women were willing to tell me. Even so, I could not agree to sending Terri onto the streets as sick as she was. And I said so.

"I agree with Carol," said one of the resident interns, to a general eye-rolling (*Oh, big surprise*) of the sobriety-and-rules crowd. "We're showing love to Terri by letting her come back. That's our mission."

"You can't expect us to follow all the rules and make the residents follow 'em but then make up new ones when you want."

I was silenced.

Suddenly Faye, who had been quiet so far, spoke up. "I don't care about enabling right now. If we don't let Terri back in here, she'll go out there and die. No one wants her, not even her mother. Only Miriam's House. She needs us."

Faye, a decade sober after many years of heroin addiction, was a strict addictions counselor. Yet she was willing, for the sake of the program we were struggling to develop, to look beyond the narrow confines of the twelve-step paradigm. Because of that and because she worked so well with the residents, Faye's word was usually definitive in these staff discussions.

We readmitted Terri. And I was so very grateful for Faye.

We managed as best we could for a few months until her addiction drove her out the door again, a repeated pattern that was to last several years. At some point after she'd gone, I could count on a phone call, usually from a hospital and just hours before a social worker called, with a plaintive voice saying, "Miss Carol, can I come home?"

And, of course, I always said yes.

For a good while it worked, in part because Terri never violated any major policy nor threatened the safety or sobriety of the community. Until, that is, together we faced what Terri and Gina did to bring it all to an end. But that wasn't until November, and in the meanwhile, they filled our house with energy and humor.

**

In the early 2000s, doctors were managing AIDS with double- and triple-therapy medications, and with drugs that treated co-occurring illnesses such as anemia, pneumonia and other lung ailments, heart problems, infections, stroke, skin rashes, and allergies. Fewer residents were dying, although we continued to admit women already in hospice care and needing a home in which to live out their final months or, in some cases, days.

Long after other people with AIDS were maintaining relative health and living more normal lives, homeless women were dying of AIDS. They were beset by poverty's effects: poor general health, erratic medication schedules due to chaotic lives or mental-health issues, and high barriers to care such as intimidating paperwork, crowded facilities with overworked staff, and inability to pay for transportation and child care. AIDS medications further damaged organs already assaulted by street drugs and alcohol. And the women who came to us tended to have a list of diseases like high blood pressure, asthma, and diabetes, and had been sick even before they contracted AIDS. So, though we worked steadily to improve our transitional program, we also admitted hospice patients and women who might never transfer out.

Between these two extremes were women who lived with us for years and women who managed only a few months. Sometimes a woman would return to us when she realized that life "out there" was just too rough and she needed to pull herself together. Several residents stayed with us long-term, meaning anywhere from eighteen months to eleven years. Kimberly was one of the first of these.

In summer of 2001, after Kimberly had been living on her own for almost a year, we heard from residents who attended the day program at Whitman Walker Clinic's Austin Center that she was losing weight and looked bad. When we contacted her, Kimberly told us her kidneys were failing, and the doctor thought she might have to start dialysis. She was depressed. We were upset. She had been doing so well, staying sober, and working her part-time job. To become ill again seemed very hard.

We readmitted Kimberly just as dialysis began. Three afternoons a week, she was picked up and taken to the dialysis center where for four hours she was attached by intravenous needles and tubes to a machine. Often when she returned home she was ill, dialysis being a process that takes blood from the body, processes it to remove waste and excess fluids, and then sends it back into the body. In doing so, it saved Kimberly's life. And it quite often made her ill, distracted, and irritable.

Yet she had also softened. Her presence in the house, when her good spirits were not bested by the unnatural process of having her blood sent out to be cleaned and returned to her by way of portals sewed into her skin, was friendlier and more accessible. She laughed and teased, she watched her horror movies. She and a new resident, Jessie, struck up an unlikely friendship that flourished despite their frequently flaring tempers. She sang what I came to think of as her signature: a low *well, well,* sliding a rough, downward glissando that managed to sound musical though it could not be considered a tune. When we heard that, we knew Kimberly was in a good mood.

We heard it most often when she'd won the lottery, which she did with a regularity that seemed to defy the odds. We could only marvel at her luck while warning her about the power of this addiction. Faye told me that she and Kimberly argued regularly about budgeting her money, mostly because Kimberly would not give up daily purchase of lottery tickets. Her strategy, not that she had thought it through, was to play the odds by playing often. When she won, it was usually ten or twenty dollars, though she did win enough larger sums—two hundred and five hundred dollars—to gain substantial notoriety around the house. With that kind of return, based on a total refusal to do some basic arithmetic about income versus expenditure, Kimberly was happy often.

Well, well.

***

When I'd opened Miriam's House, I had expected that AIDS and the other illnesses besetting our residents would be the prime issues, the most tragic and the least amenable to improvement. But as I watched the effects of alcohol and drug abuse on women who had showed strength, character, and spirit before relapsing, I began to think of addictions as, if not more important, then at least as urgent as AIDS. You couldn't witness the shame and defeat on the faces of women who'd relapsed, nor see how previously bright and engaging personalities changed for the worse, nor attend funerals of those whose relapse had killed them, without pondering the vicious connection between AIDS and addictions.

So Tim and I took very seriously that we were living in a clean and sober community. We brought no alcohol into our apartment, not even for cooking, and we never drank when we were out and about in Washington. Our strict sobriety symbolized solidarity with the women and a way to participate more fully in the life and struggles of the community we loved. This was to us a natural and even obvious choice, so much so that we had no idea how strange or even unnecessary it might seem to other people. When, in 2000, our board of directors, packed with new and eager faces, proposed a grand gala complete with open bar, we were completely unprepared for it. And they were completely unprepared for our resistance.

***

The relationship between a nonprofit's founding executive director and her board of directors is a strange one. Technically, the board owns and is ultimately in charge of the organization. It supervises the executive director, or CEO, who is directly responsible to the board. It's an ill-defined combination of trusting, supporting, and supervising the executive in a way that doesn't interfere with day-to-day management—a tricky balance that must be understood and kept by both parties. Even in the best situation, the relationship can be fraught with differing understandings of roles and limits, and by conflicting ideals for the organization and its mission.

As the founder of Miriam's House, I had dreamed of, fought for, brought to pass, and was managing this thing that was both deeply personal and the pinnacle of my professional aspirations. By 2001, half of the board members had not known me or Miriam's House before their recruitment onto the board. The president, Kathy, and I had wanted to avoid the more typical model of the insular board comprising only friends and other like-minded nonprofit leaders and volunteers. So in 1999 we'd begun recruiting outside our usual circles and found a couple persons of wealth, two women with MBAs, and a man with extensive experience in the business world. It seemed ideal to have a board that included the like-minded *and* the broadening influences. And those were precisely the lines along which the board fell apart in June of 2001.

Tim and I set up the eventual rift when we resisted a proposal by the mover-and-shaker board members for a fancy gala. We were leery of taking on anything so complicated. We knew, and rightly so, as it turned out, that a lot of work would devolve upon us despite the members' protestations they'd keep that from happening. Tim, as a professional fundraiser, knew how hard it was and how long it took to make annual galas successful. And the newer members of the board seemed to be inordinately sensitive about how they were treated and whether they had our unquestioning compliance. We, unused to and even impatient with their easily bruised egos and need for deference, would go only so far to appease them. Finally, the foil for all this became the question of alcohol.

You can't have a gala fundraiser without alcohol, was the position of half the board members, the ones planning for and excited about the function. You can't have alcohol at a function for a clean-and-sober house, was the position of Tim and me and the original and like-minded board members. The twain threatened never to meet until we agreed on a compromise: a two-part gala with no alcohol at the reception and concert, to which residents and their families were invited, then dinner at which alcohol would be served and to which the residents and their families were not invited.

But even though the event went well and the compromise turned out to be a good one, the stage had been set for a divide that, through inattention, we allowed to widen to an icy crevasse into which all hope of agreement and compromise fell and disappeared. Gradually, and in spite of the fact that my performance evaluations had always been excellent, certain individuals began displaying mounting discontent with my work and disrespect for me. The treasurer, whose role it was to take responsibility for and present quarterly financial reports, instead spent forty-five minutes of board meetings harassing Tim and me about one or two line items. An MBA-holder took it upon herself to question my supervisory abilities and offer unsolicited advice. Planning for another gala became a focal point for argument, and the question of alcohol on which it all hinged became a convenient vehicle for expressing the resentments and anger about everything we weren't talking about: money, class, and entitlement.

Finally, in May of 2001, just after the treasurer announced she was moving to another state, two board members resigned. A third joined them, although not before he'd sent a group e-mail calling me facetious and listing all the ways in which I was an incompetent leader. To underscore the point, the treasurer also handed in a resignation, completely unnecessary in light of her previous letter citing her pending move and pointedly marking her solidarity with the rest of the defectors.

Desperate and feeling like a total failure, I called Valerie.

Her point of view—*You know, they could have fired you*—perversely helped me feel a little better about the whole debacle. I had survived a coup, and my sense was that they, discontent as they were, could actually make no case for my incompetence and removal.

It was tempting to reject the defectors as privileged snobs who just didn't understand our mission. But Miriam's House had established too strong a reliance on honesty and openness. So we remaining board members wrestled with how and why our experiment in balancing the experience, knowledge, and economic status of members had gone so badly awry. We worked with Valerie for six months until we had a revised recruitment plan, officer job descriptions, and greater clarity on how to share our mission. We set about recruiting new members.

In all this, we had the model of the residents, whom we asked to commit to the hard work of recovery from addiction, bad habits, suddenly useless survival strategies, and negative thinking. *If we expect the women to do it, we have to be able to do it ourselves,* I wrote in my journal.

I reflected that here was yet another struggle between people, only these people had been the same race as me. It wasn't always black and white. It was also economic. It was class. And I was dealing with just one of those social pitfalls. The women I served and loved were dealing with all three, a triple whammy the blows of which they had to dodge or absorb every single day.

**

The board rebellion, coming as it did on top of the job that I often feared I was mucking up, shook me deeply. I needed a break. A serious break, not just a long weekend. That spring, while the board fell apart around me, I investigated month-long retreats. By some happy circumstance and despite my utter ignorance of such matters, I discovered a Jesuit Center in Wernersville, Pennsylvania, with a July silent retreat based on something called the Ignatian Spiritual Exercises. Lifelong Protestant that I was, I knew nothing of Catholics and their ways, but the thought of thirty days in silence so appealed to me that, cheerfully unaware, I applied. Once accepted, I thought it best to educate myself at least a bit, which I did by checking in with a couple of Catholic friends.

In the meanwhile, there was an organization to run, and nothing stopped just because I was going through trauma with my board and dreaming of thirty blissful days talking to no one. Life at Miriam's House persisted in careening dizzily from the sublime to the ridiculous. Jackee was incontinent but often refused to wear adult diapers because, as she said—and so truly that no one could muster a persuasive argument—they made her look fat. When we went to Kennedy Center to hear my sister, Joan, perform with her flute-and-harp duo, I kept nervously looking to see if Jackee's chair was dripping. Meanwhile, Kimberly fell to making snide comments about Jackee that she insisted were to herself but that, since she made them aloud, in the dining room, deep voiced, became bait that Jackee was constitutionally unable to ignore. We had to make sure they were not sitting near one another at the celebratory party for a resident's graduation from her treatment program. Terri's eyesight was failing, and she'd been discharged from yet another program due to poor health. Gina wasn't speaking to me because I'd put the chicken she was thawing on the counter (against oft-repeated food-handling policy) into the refrigerator. Ruby, admitted under hospice care a few weeks before, was dying and seemed to be the only resident at peace. At a retirement party for one of the nurses, Terri told me she wanted to move to a different room because her corner room tended to be colder than others. But when I suggested Nickie's old room, she said, loudly enough for everyone else to hear, that she wouldn't go near that room. Then pointedly ignoring my equally pointed refusal to ask what she meant, she rambled on about them big smelly bags Nickie used to drag out of there like she was disposing of heaps of body parts, and I could be sure that she (Terri) would never move into the body-parts room.

And yet, I could tell my work with Valerie was still paying off. Life was simpler, work was easier when I relied upon Donna's ability to handle any crisis, and I admitted that Faye and I actually could get along and that she was really wise. I stayed quiet while Yvonne, increasingly self-confident, shared her insights at staff meeting. I sought out Elsie for lovely discussions about addictions and spirituality. I remembered to rely on Tim's successful fundraising and unfailing support from behind the scenes. And we had four interns that summer, so my only regular duty shifts were on Monday evenings. Such unprecedented riches allowed me more rest and personal time that summer of 2001 than I'd had since we opened five years before.

***

In early August, I sat on a wood bench overlooking the long drive from the entrance of the retreat center in Wernersville. So I had sat during the past month on other benches and in other hushed spaces of those acres of woods, corn fields, paths, tiny woodland shrines, and quiet, quiet days. But this was my final day, and I was waiting to catch a first glimpse of our car. Tim and I had never in the eight years of our marriage been apart for so long.

"Go gently," Sister Susan Marie, the spiritual director with whom I met every day of the thirty-day exercises, would say at the end of each session. Perhaps she said it because she sensed how anxiety could drive me, perhaps she said it to everyone she was directing. No matter, it became something of a mantra in the years ahead.

"Let me stay quiet for a while," I said after Tim and I had hugged, retrieved the luggage from my room, roamed around for picture-taking, and then set out on the four-hour drive home to DC. "It's been so peaceful, so beautiful here, and I want to hold onto that feeling before getting back into the city, back to work." Tim nodded and drove in silence for a long while.

When I finally was ready to hear about work and home he told me about Rebecca, who had moved in while I was on retreat.

"She had a stroke a year ago that completely incapacitated her, so she stays in a wheelchair or in bed. She can't talk, speech aphasia I think it's called, and she also has trouble swallowing. Her emotions are right out in the open, I think that's a result of the stroke, too. She cries or laughs at the drop of a hat. And she understands everything, she really observes us."

He told me how the PCAs cared for her, made all her meals and helped her feed herself, bathed and changed and dressed her in the morning, and undressed her at night. Aside from dying women, we had never admitted a resident who needed so much care.

"But she's already a part of the family," Tim said.

Soon after I arrived at Miriam's House, unpacked my bags, and started a load of wash, I went to Rebecca's room to introduce myself. Her door was propped open so staff could easily keep an eye on her. Not wanting to startle her, I stopped to look in before speaking.

Rebecca sat in her wheelchair in front of the television, drooping forward and leaning to one side. In her neatly combed and platted hair I thought I detected the loving hand of a certain PCA. She was dressed in jeans and a buttoned shirt. A long, slender string of saliva, glistening in the light from the window behind her, connected her mouth to her white shirt just below its pointed collar. The drool cloth, loosely held in her hands, rested on her lap. Was she asleep? I made a slight sound. She looked up.

"May I come in?" I went in when she grunted, moving her right arm in a barely controlled gesture. Over the noise of the television, I said, "Hi, Rebecca. I'm Carol. I'm Tim's wife. I live here, too, and work in the office."

She lifted her head, slowly, clumsily, as though it were too heavy or her neck too weak. Her eyes, gray and aware, fixed on me. She gave what I later told Tim could only be described as a chortle.

"I know you can't speak," I said, and I knelt down at her side. "May I?" I gestured toward the drool cloth. She nodded, another heavily awkward movement of her neck. I picked up the cloth to clean the saliva on her mouth and shirt. Still under the influence of my own days of silence, I added that God speaks through us best when we don't talk, anyway.

When she immediately coughed a couple of wet sobs I wondered if I'd said the wrong thing, kneeling at her side and wiping the tears and saliva and snot from her face. But she quickly calmed and returned her attention to the TV, so I left. *Go gently.*

The next time I saw Rebecca was at house meeting on Tuesday afternoon. Linda, the PCA who had already staked a claim as Rebecca's especial companion and aide, and whose hand I had indeed detected in the platted hair, wheeled her into the circle and took a chair next to her after making sure the drool cloth was handy and Rebecca was comfortable.

"Hello, Rebecca. You're looking snazzy." She chortled at me, then looked down at the bright yellow capris with a knife-sharp crease, matching yellow socks, and white sliders. She chortled again, plucking at the blue-yellow-white plaid shirt.

"She's trying to say she have a new shirt." Linda leaned over to gently apply the drool cloth to what had been released by the chortles. "I found it downstairs in the donations box."

I knew Linda. She hadn't just found a shirt. She had chosen it carefully from among the other donated clothing, made sure it matched the pants, then washed and ironed the ensemble.

After we all had admired Rebecca's outfit, we began house meeting as usual, going around the circle so each person had a chance to share highs and lows, or, if not wanting to share, passing it on. After staff business and announcements, a couple of the women began one of those convoluted and complaint-filled conversations that happened semiregularly, obsessing over some item of safety or sanitation or food theft. I had developed the habit of allowing the main points to be aired twice, but by the third time around I always stepped in. As I was opening my mouth to do just that, Rebecca began to shake. Puzzled, I stopped and looked across the circle at her. She swayed in her chair, head bobbing, entire body quivering so she could not manage even her habitual slumping posture. Collapsing at the waist, face pointed at her lap, she laughed.

The saliva poured from her mouth. She watched it puddle onto the brightly clean pants, glanced up at Linda's face and laughed harder. She reached for the drool cloth and directed it toward her mouth. But the laughter-induced quaking messed up her aim and the cloth dabbed at her ear instead, eliciting another wail of full-bodied glee.

What could we do? We laughed with her, closed the meeting with no further complaints, and stood up for what ended every single meeting at Miriam's House. We put arms around shoulders or grabbed hands. Linda took Rebecca's right wrist (the hand held the drool-soaked towel) and the resident to her other side had put a hand on her left shoulder. Rebecca's face was still.

Lord, grant me the serenity to accept the things I cannot change, the courage to change the things that I can, and the wisdom to know the difference.

And then Linda wheeled Rebecca to the dining room to place her at her favorite spot, from which she could see what was happening in the kitchen and still monitor dining-room conversations. There she would stay until her meal was cooked and fed to her, spoonful by spoonful, Linda wiping from her chin the food that oozed over it, threatening to drip down and ruin the pretty new shirt.

CHAPTER TWENTY-TWO

I was on duty one evening in November 2001 when a resident came to me and said she smelled beer at the end of the first-floor hallway. There were few things I dreaded hearing more than this. Using alcohol or drugs in the house was addressed with the most severe penalty on our books: immediately beginning discharge procedures. This was our one no-compromise rule. In a community of women trying to kick their addictions, the presence of drugs or alcohol was extremely threatening. No resident had a right to make recovery so difficult for the rest.

With growing alarm, then, I walked down the first-floor residents' hall, sniffing. The smell was strongest outside Terri's door. But Terri had been ill, was just returned from the hospital and barely able to make it from her room to the dining room. She hadn't left the house for days. She couldn't have anything in there.

Unsure, I sniffed again. Yes. I knocked at her door. She called me in.

"Terri, I smell alcohol." I could form no more words. Terri froze, curled up on the bed, all watchful brown eyes, fragile bone, and wary stillness. I began to look around. I checked under the bed, on the dresser, in the bathroom, at the window. We didn't speak. Except for those following eyes, she didn't move.

The room was a mess. I searched through the piles of clothing on floor and chair, discarded snack bags, and refuse from hospital stays—plastic pitchers and kidney-shaped plastic bowls, stacks of medical papers. Just as I straightened up from looking under the bed I saw it, the beer can, sitting on top of the pile in her small trashcan, semihidden between the headboard and the bedside table. Without looking at Terri, I reached for it. I had to go to my office. I turned away with the can, holding it gingerly between two fingers and away from my body as though it were a coiled snake.

Still, she was still.

I left her. I had to write the incident report. Best to get it done right away.

Not until much later, after finishing the incident report, after she had agreed to stay in her room until meeting with Yvonne and me in the morning, and after I was in my apartment in bed and not asleep, did the question arise. Who had brought that beer into the house for her?

The next morning Yvonne and I, after consulting with Faye, planned for our meeting with Terri. Over the years, we had developed two kinds of special meetings with residents: the compassion meeting and the staffing. The former had a cautionary yet supportive message: we see a pattern developing that concerns us and we want to check in with and hear from you. A compassion meeting had a *let's work together on this* feel. The latter was stern, usually coming after a serious violation of policy or a series of smaller actions that added up to bigger trouble.

This meeting with Terri went beyond even a staffing. This was not about a pattern, this was about the violation of our one bottom-line rule. This meeting was to inform her that we were beginning discharge procedures. And we needed to know how she got the beer.

My role in discharge meetings was to be the bad cop, authoritarian yet fair, the one with the message about how discharge works, what her rights were, and how she could access the ombudsman office to protest the decision or get counseling. The good-cop role belonged to the other staff member at the meeting and functioned as the softer voice in the room, offering emotional support and promising help through the entire ordeal. Yvonne was to be the good cop, and we met in the staff lounge to prepare for the meeting.

"Why? Why would she do something so stupid?"

"It's not about why, Carol, and you know we got to do this. She's got no right to upset the others who are trying to stay clean. I just can't believe it's ending like this after all we been through with her."

I thought about the many times in and out of treatment, stretching our rules, all the promises to be good.

Yvonne reached for the discharge papers I'd placed on the table in front of me. I stared out the window, which looked into a window well. The ground floor was half below grade, so the view from the two windows in the staff lounge was a concrete wall and a cheerless gray sky. Yvonne pushed the papers back across the table. "Well, I know we should find out how that beer got into the house. She sure didn't run out to buy it with her weak, sick self."

Terri knocked on the door and we called her in. As she took her seat I tried not to notice how large she made the chair look. She sat perched forward, back straight, and Terri— contentious, amusing, verbal, quick-witted Terri—said nothing.

She nodded as I explained why I had the discharge papers ready. She leaned forward slightly to look attentively at each sheet as I placed it before her and explained what it meant. She accepted the pen in her little hand with its lank, long fingers and signed where I indicated.

Brown eyes huge in her gaunt face, she nodded at Yvonne's promise of support and help. Finally she spoke.

"I'm sorry, Miss Carol. I'm sorry, Miss Yvonne."

I had the thought that it might have been easier if she'd died, and I had been through enough at Miriam's House not to be shocked at myself for thinking it.

"Terri," Yvonne said gently, "we need to know how you got the beer."

"No." Terri would not be persuaded to tell us how that beer got into Miriam's House. We suspected she was protecting another resident, though we didn't know whom. But there could be few secrets in a community like Miriam's House, and most that did exist didn't remain in the dark for long. Within a few days of the meeting with Terri the women were restless and angry. They knew who was getting away with buying and bringing in the beer, and their sense of fairness, always strong, rebelled. They requested an emergency meeting.

We convened our community meetings in the living room. Like the dining room, with which it formed an L-shaped space, the room had a bay of large windows and a capacious feel. Also similar to the dining room, it saw a lot of life: house meetings, workshops, parties, memorial services. And emergency meetings, sometimes called by staff, sometimes by residents. For this one, I got to the living room early and arranged the chairs and sofas in a circle. Then I sat there alone, waiting in the quiet, wanting to be calm and centered for what was ahead.

They came in slowly, morosely, dropping onto the soft cushions of the sofa, draping sideways in the chairs, staring at the floor. No one took pleasure in what was about to happen. This was not about vindictiveness, this was about justice and recovery. We dispensed with the usual check-in. I looked around at the upset and angry women, took a slow breath and asked, "Who wants to begin?"

"It ain't fair, Miss Carol. We know Terri has to leave, but someone brought her that beer. And she should have to leave, too."

"Yeah, she just as bad to be around here as Terri."

"It ain't fair unless Gin . . . the other one go, too."

My mouth went dry. *Good Lord, not Gina.* But I didn't know who I'd rather it be.

"You know," I said, "if we're going to talk about another resident, she should be here."

Someone went to rouse her from her room. Her health had been deteriorating, and she'd been sleeping a lot while not at the doctor's office or in the emergency room. When Gina dragged in, she took the nearest chair, slumped over her lap, and stared at the hands she picked at.

"Gina, your friends have something to say to you." I nodded encouragement I did not feel to the women around her.

Gina, confronted by the wrathful accusations of her peers, admitted the truth.

Life sometimes presents one with impossible choices that are ambiguous in all but one respect: a choice must be made. Out of Miriam's House they went, first Terri and then Gina. Terri somehow persuaded her mother to let her move back home, which was a relief in one way, a concern in another. That neighborhood did not seem to be the wisest place for Terri to live, given that she had a lot of longtime drinking buddies there. But we had no alternatives, so we helped her move.

Once Terri was housed we could concentrate on the much more difficult placement for Gina, who had thoroughly alienated family members during her drugging years. Six weeks passed before we found a place for her. Her uncle, long a favorite of Gina's, finally agreed to let her live with him in Silver Spring, Maryland. I drove Gina up Georgia Avenue one morning in December.

As we pulled her bags and boxes from the back of the van, I looked around and was relieved to see that the tiny house was in good repair and the yard well kept. Her uncle showed us in, gesturing to the sofa on which she would sleep in the tidy, sparsely furnished living room. We put her bags down, and I tried not to worry about the lack of privacy. Residents had gone to worse places, had come from worse places. I felt a measure of peace in my heart as I climbed into the van and drove away.

But still I had to pull over once out of sight of the house when tears prevented me from seeing where I was going.

***

She was the first of a handful of Caucasian woman we welcomed to Miriam's House. I remember wondering how it would work, whether we would be dealing with racial or cultural tensions, given that all the other residents were African or African American. But I didn't yet know Claudia, and I was underestimating the generosity of the women.

I have a photo of her, sitting in the dining room with a smile so big her eyes crinkle up and just about disappear. She might have been comical, especially as she had no compunction about that smile revealing toothless gums, except for the joy that scintillated around her. Any worries about racial tensions receded by the end of her first day with us because Claudia welcomed all with her signature cheer, conflict included.

She moved in during November 2001, a medium-build, cheerful woman, her hair spiking reddish wisps above the beaming face and her outfit mismatched as though she were color-blind. Her possessions were few because she had been either homeless or institutionalized most of her life. But little seemed to matter to Claudia aside from her drum, a beautiful instrument that looked to be African in the Djembe style. She blithely told us she was a drummer, and we took that in the professional sense because she was so sure of herself. She offered to keep the drum in the living room so others could use it, and we imagined group drumming lessons. With some excitement, a few residents and staff gathered in the living room the next night after dinner to hear Claudia play.

She sat at the drum, radiating pride, lifted her hands, bowed her head, and began pounding. And pounding. We could discern no rhythm, no indication of a pattern, nothing musical except the look of ecstasy on Claudia's face. We applauded madly when she was done, cheering and standing up to clap her on the back. She again offered to teach us, and we had our first lesson then and there.

It seemed perfect that a woman of such happiness would be with us over a Christmas season, the sole holiday during her short stay. Tim took that photograph during our annual holiday party. Visible in it are the poinsettia tablecloth and a red-and-green popcorn tin decorated with snowmen. Claudia wears a bulky white sweater with gold and red trim at the shoulders and down the bodice. She does look odd, with the huge grin innocent of any teeth at all and cheek muscles so vigorously engaged that her eyes are barely visible. Even a cursory glance at her would correctly tell you that she was mentally ill, but as with all of our residents, Claudia deserved better than cursory. And yet it is easy to dismiss the Claudias of the world.

I know because I did.

We'd had a conversation on the day the photo was taken. I was on a break from the party preparations, sitting in the dining room and listening to Christmas music when Claudia came in.

"Oh, I love this!" She was referring to the carol playing at that moment. She halted, clasped her hands under her chin, and closed her eyes, swaying. Claudia had a decided flair for the dramatic in her stories and demeanor. As the carol ended, she came out of her trance and sat at the table with me. "You know, I sang that in a choir. Who's singing?"

"The Mormon Tabernacle Choir."

"Yes, the Mormon Tabernacle Choir."

I stared.

She said she'd also sung Handel's *Messiah* with them.

Claudia was Mormon? Oh yes, she had sung with them for twenty-five years when she lived out west. Just after graduating from the music college, of course.

I didn't like to dismiss out of hand what I was being told, but . . . Mormon? *College?*

Yes, and she had been a ballerina. The swan in *Swan Lake.* She had toured all over the world. That was after the Mormon Tabernacle Choir. They toured, too. She had been to Russia and Egypt and Kenya.

Claudia's guileless eyes met mine.

"Oh, Claudia, what a wonderful life you've had." At that point, I mentally checked out of the conversation, my mind wandering to my apartment kitchen and the turkey I needed to run upstairs to baste. I could sit for a few minutes while Claudia invented implausible tales, but pretty soon it would be time to escape. Nodding vaguely and *hmmm*-ing some more while she went on about something else, I turned my thoughts to more important matters like that unbasted turkey and the fact that the house would be full of guests in a few hours.

When I did finally allow Claudia to capture my respectful attention, it was on the night she died.

As long as I lived and worked with women living with AIDS, the sudden slide into death of one who had seemed well always left me dazed. In some strange way I would forget that she was ill, would somehow discount the severity of the diagnosis. As I lived with these women, sharing life with them and loving them, I think I began to believe we would all live forever.

Such was the case with Claudia. Not long after telling her stories of life as a professional chorister and prima ballerina, she was in George Washington Hospital with liver failure. We'd barely had time to adjust to this before we were told that she had less than a month to live. Death from liver failure, her doctors said, needed more nursing capability than we had, so she was admitted to a nursing home for hospice care. We arranged a visit as soon as her caregivers allowed it. Five residents and I got ready to visit her one wintery January evening.

"Give Claudia a kiss for me!"

"Wait. Don't she like stuffed bears? We got to bring a stuffed bear."

"I got a extra bear. Be right back."

"What, now we waiting for Kimberly to get a bear? Getting hot in this coat."

"Elsie, shouldn't they take a plate? I got some pigs feet and biscuits and . . ."

"No, not on this first visit, not until we know what her diet is."

"Here come Kimberly. Carol, put the gospel station in the van."

And so we headed out, six of us, stepping around icy patches on the sidewalk and shivering in the van until it warmed up enough to kick out some heat. The nursing home was not far, just over on Wisconsin Avenue, and so the trip lasted barely long enough for belting out a couple of gospel songs as accompaniment to the radio.

Claudia's room was near the nursing station, which occupied the center of a ring with the patient rooms on the perimeter. We found her sitting up in the bed, propped by several pillows, face haggard. Yet the smile with which she greeted us was just as brilliant as ever. As we hugged and well-wished and relayed messages she reached for the teddy bear and hugged it to her chest.

"I had the most beautiful dream!" Frail and shining, Claudia leaned toward us over the bear clasped in her lap, its fuzzy round ears framing her chin. The room was fairly large and Claudia its only occupant. Her window, etched in frost, looked into a courtyard shrouded in drifts of snow. The winter evening lay serenely beyond, vigilant.

"I was asleep but not asleep. And there was an angel, a beautiful angel, all in white and gold and shiny. She filled the sky. And there was a tear on her face. But not a tear of sorrow. A tear of joy."

We left her fifteen minutes later in an uncharacteristic silence that lasted through the ride back to Miriam's House. I ate some supper, then went to check in with Elsie. On my way past the kitchen, I heard Kimberly telling about Claudia's angel dream. After a quick conversation with Elsie, I got back into the van and, three hours after we had left her room, walked back into it. I had learned on the earlier visit that the nurses estimated Claudia had fewer than twenty-four hours left. Even though these guesses usually turned out to be wrong, I wanted to make good our promise to her that she would not die alone. Someone could come take my place if she made it to the morning.

And there I stayed through the peaceful night, my back to the window with its crystalline tracings and facing Claudia, who was unconscious and had been so, a nurse told me, since shortly after we'd left her. One of the nurses at N Street Village, the women's shelter and program where Claudia had stayed before she came to us, visited for a while. Occasionally a nurse entered, checked her pulse and breathing, nodded at me, and left. Several times an aide came in to apply gel to her chapped lips, run a moist swab around her parched mouth, and turn her in the bed.

Otherwise I was alone, there with Claudia, her dream, the onyx night, and my thoughts about turkeys and parties and stories bubbling up through mental illness's porous filters, unheeded by the careless listener. Occasionally I smoothed lotion on her hands and arms and chatted quietly about goings-on back home. Once I rearranged pillows discommoded in her sole bout of restlessness. At around three o'clock, she coughed and gagged. I jumped over to her, grabbed her shoulders, and turned her on her side. Dark crimson vomit flowed over the sheets and onto the floor. I found a care aide and told her. She looked at me significantly, cleaned up the vomit, and said as she left, "It's good you're here."

After that, Claudia returned to the peaceful state that had marked the entire night. So still was she that I worried I might fall asleep, that she might die while I was not awake and present to her. I stood to gaze out onto the pristine, drifted snow in the courtyard beyond the window. I massaged more lotion into her hands. She was so calm.

Close to five o'clock, as I was planning to call Miriam's House to arrange for another staff member to come and sit with Claudia, she coughed lightly. I looked up. The muscles at her clavicle pulled tight and released. She gasped. I moved swiftly to the bed to position myself behind her, propping her up a bit and with my arms around her. She gasped again, her neck's sinew and cord distended. I lay my cheek on her head

and whispered. *We love you. We all love you. You're so beautiful. Go home to God.* She gasped and gasped again. Then she
was perfectly still.

Claudia: precious, odd, holy. Claudia of the dream. Claudia
who had deserved better of me.

CHAPTER TWENTY-THREE

Rebecca lived with us for eighteen months, from July 2001 to February 2003, a time period that included the death of a young woman whose circumstances were only slightly less tragic than Alyssa's had been. Gina returned for more dining-room dancing and ER dramas before her death, and we admitted Jessie, whose seven-year stay with us was to be marked by her struggles with depression and fear, and my fight to keep her at Miriam's House. But Rebecca's story comes first, if only because the way she lived and died deserves attention all its own.

***

Rebecca, for all she could be volatile and impatient, received special care from staff. Linda, the PCA who had taken Rebecca under her wing as soon as she moved in, made sure her room was spruced up and held homey touches that Rebecca couldn't manage herself, like photos, flowers, and doilies. Linda found cute outfits for Rebecca and was always her personal attendant on house outings to the theater or Six Flags.

She still required a lot of staff attention, and just as we'd settled into a workable routine with her, one of our PCAs needed medical leave. Yvonne told me about it at a team meeting in the spring. "The leave will be at least six weeks. The other personal-care aides are already covering a lot of extra hours because of their vacations. We have to cover the night shift some way."

We had always had trouble finding someone willing to work part time and temporarily. Besides, we were so particular about our staff and how they related to the residents that we knew we'd only just be starting to trust a new PCA when the other would be ready to come back. That would be a large investment for little return. Most important, it would be hard on Rebecca to be cared for by a stranger who then left her just as she was getting used to her.

So we resorted to a solution we'd established some years ago for nights when we'd been short staffed. I would take the house's mobile phone—the one always carried by a PCA or intern on duty after office hours and on weekends—warn the residents not to call after eleven o'clock except for emergencies, post a sign reminding them, and lock the kitchen door for safety. Yvonne suggested I ask the resident interns to take some shifts, but I didn't like to do that, telling her theirs was already an intense and often difficult year. "We'll do what we've done before. We'll put up the sign, lock the kitchen, and tell Rebecca that I'm her help for the night. I'll just sleep until she calls."

Yvonne said she would cover some daytime or evening shifts herself in order to free up PCAs to take a couple of the night shifts. That would leave me with three or four nights a week instead of five or seven. And so for the next six weeks I was regularly on call for Rebecca, sleeping with the house phone on my bedside table.

***

The phone rang and I dragged myself awake, trying to answer before Tim, asleep beside me, was disturbed. The number was on speed dial on Rebecca's phone, and she knew I'd be the one to answer on these nights without a PCA available.

She didn't speak, of course, but there was the familiar gurgling laugh when I mumbled into the phone. We had done this often enough for me to tease her. Rebecca loved trash talk.

"Why the hell are you bothering me now? It's two o'clock in the morning. Can't you leave me alone?"

I waited for the belly laugh, then told Rebecca to give me a minute to get dressed and downstairs. The house was still except for the faint sounds of the women's radios and televisions. I paused a moment at the large window on the second-floor staircase landing, loving how the cherry trees' newly budding branches looked in the street lamps' pallid light. I grinned as I went downstairs to the first floor and into the residents' hallway, listening for the chortle that signaled she'd heard me coming.

She was lying amidst a tangle of sheets and pillows, quilt half off the bed. Looked like a restless night.

"Hey, Rebecca. Need a change?"

She nodded, a ponderous swing of her head. I pulled the tangle of sheets aside and out of the way. Rebecca reached for the bed rail with her one good arm, the right one, pulling herself onto her left side and holding steady while I placed an absorbent pad beneath her and tucked a folded edge of it under her body like the PCAs taught me. She grunted with the effort of resisting my yank at the tape on the diaper. After I'd tugged it free of her hips, she let go of the rail and fell back. I reached around, one hand under her shoulder, the other under her hip, *one-two-three*, and rolled her onto her right side. She braced herself, left arm crooked in front of her chest, elbow pressed against the mattress. I smoothed the pad flat on the far side, loosened the tape, and pushed the diaper free of her hips and as far down her buttocks as I could. Immediately she flopped onto her back, and I pulled the diaper, then rolled it and threw it into the red medical-waste bag.

Sometimes we exchanged words and grunts, but mostly we were quiet except for the sounds of Rebecca's patient, heavy breathing, and the water sloshing in the basin. The routine was familiar and comforting—Rebecca's mute acceptance of the intimacy, the cleansing of skin with soapy water and sweet-smelling lotion, the clean diaper snugly fitted around her hips, the satisfaction of a tidy bed and the comfort of another pillow or a sip of ice water, the leave-taking with Rebecca already falling asleep.

The house peaceful around us, I headed upstairs to my apartment.

***

The ill PCA returned in early summer 2002, and glad as I was for the uninterrupted nights, I felt as though I'd lost something precious. The humble service I'd offered Rebecca seemed a pure expression of the intent of my life and work at Miriam's House.

So much of what I did was a step or two removed from the daily life of the residents. The job of the executive director is not to involve herself in the minutiae of her charges' lives, and I had set myself clear boundaries so as not to interfere with the work of other staff or set myself up with an authority I did not have. But what gave me real joy, apart from those lovely lists of checked-off tasks in my daily planner, was relating on an intimate level with the residents. As I grew freer of needing to be liked and to hoard every scrap of approval I could get, I reveled in the deepening connections and the sense that these women who seemed so different from me were, actually, not so different after all.

And so being in *service* to was gradually transformed into being *present* to. It changed into a kind of companionship that, while never in denial about the very real status differential between us, made for an easy camaraderie of reciprocity rather than always a giving/receiving exchange in which I had all the power. All the while, that giving and receiving was happening, obviously. But there was transformation in changing an adult's diapers and learning to do it lovingly, without ego or hidden agenda. There was transformation in a helpless woman's acceptance of intimacies that one hopes never to have to suffer oneself. There was humility in ceasing to help the vulnerable and commencing to be with them. To stay with them.

***

The community had taken Rebecca into its heart. We gathered around her hoping to make her laugh. We figured out what she was trying to say when she pointed out pictures or words in the little communication book an intern had made for her. We tried to interpret her gestures, though Linda was the only one who could do that with any accuracy, saying "She want one of them popsicles," or "She need a change," when all I could perceive were random arm movements. I loved seeing Linda and Rebecca together, as theirs was a special bond. So when Linda told me she was going to Six Flags amusement park with seven women and the interns, and she was getting together special outfits for Rebecca and her, I couldn't wait to see how they looked.

On the day of the trip, I ran out to the front patio to see the group off. Planning for it had been an exercise in organized frustration, what with the logistical nightmares of two wheelchairs, two cars for eleven people, Rebecca who was incontinent and needed lots of supplies, and providing lunch because the food in the park was so expensive. I wanted to check with the interns and women before they left. But most of all I wanted to see Rebecca and Linda in their outfits.

"Linda! Wait!"

She stopped rolling the wheelchair and turned around. "Oh, there you are, Carol. We couldn't find you."

"I know, and I just have to check you two out before you go."

Rebecca chortled and waved her right arm toward Linda, then at herself, *ahhhhhh*. Linda wore a yellow top, white capris, white sandals, and a white cap. Rebecca wore a white top, yellow capris, white sandals, and a white cap.

"Wow, Rebecca, you and Linda will be the best dressed in the park," I said, bending down to give her a kiss on the forehead before turning to Linda with a thank-you pat on the arm. "Make sure you get a picture, okay?"

They were gone most of the day. I was at my desk when I heard the front door open and the voices, raucous, arguing companionably about who felt sickest on the roller coasters and who got wettest on the water rides. I went out to the lobby as the main group passed and Rebecca and Linda came up on the elevator. I stared.

"Rebecca, where's your other sandal?"

She was wearing only the right one. Her left foot was bare. *Ahhhhhh!* She waved her right arm at her left foot and looked up at Linda while laughing hard enough to choke. Linda clapped her on the back. "Easy, girl." But she, too, laughed as Rebecca held up the bare foot and gestured again for Linda to tell the story.

"It fell off into the water at one of them rides where you splash downhill and get going so fast. Before we knew it, no shoe! Rebecca, calm down. Don't be choking like that."

Rebecca, bare foot stuck out in front of her, couldn't stop laughing. I slipped back into my office while Linda took Rebecca to her room to settle her down and clean her up. Later the next week, Linda gave the photograph I'd asked for. In it, the two of them smiled from under their white caps, perfectly dressed except for that one bare foot. I framed it and Tim put it up on the kitchen hallway wall that now bore a five-year photographic record of life at Miriam's House.

***

Not long after this, Rebecca began to decline physically. Elsie and Linda raised their concerns at a staff meeting during the summer of 2002, just about the time of the one-year marker for Rebecca's admission to Miriam's House.

"When she came to us, she could eat pretty well. But now she choke a lot and I'm plain scared to feed her. She sound like she about to die."

"And if I feed her after Yvonne has gone for the day, I got no one to really help me if something happens."

I was really grateful that the PCAs had managed for as long and as well as they had, and I told them so. "I can hardly sit at the table with her. I like to think of myself as a compassionate person, but the sight of Rebecca with the slobber and food dripping out of her mouth is just too much. Sometimes I have to leave the dining room or else I'll throw up."

We had recently begun preparing her food differently when we noticed she was choking more easily. We cooked the heck out of it and then swirled it in the blender so that what was on the plate looked quite a bit like baby food, only less appetizing.

Poor Rebecca hated that blenderized food. Linda reported Rebecca crying and closing her mouth when the spoon was put to her lips.

This made Elsie scoff and say that Linda had got off easy. "Last night she swung that one good arm at the plate and knocked it clear out of my hands. Spilled all over the floor, table, and me. Had to clean it up and then cook more."

Yvonne thought for a moment. "I don't know about cooking more if she does that again. We can't let her be treating us like that. Next time, let her go hungry."

We agreed that the fair way to do this was to warn her in advance. Yvonne was delegated to have this conversation with Rebecca the next day. She also said she'd call Rebecca's doctor. Staff meeting ended and we stood up as usual, put arms around one another, and recited the Serenity Prayer.

Later that fall, Yvonne asked me into her office to tell me Rebecca's doctor had called after seeing Rebecca for a routine checkup the day before. Glumly, she told me that the doctor wanted to surgically insert a stomach tube through which we would feed a liquid supplement directly into her stomach.

"Oh no. The poor woman can't even wipe her own behind, and now she won't be able to eat? That's just torture—everyone else is cooking and eating, and she's sitting there waiting for Boost to be funneled into her stomach."

"I know." Yvonne repeated what the doctor had said, that because Rebecca was choking on even the softest foods it seemed she had lost most of her swallowing function. Plus she was not getting much nutrition, and there was the danger of food particles getting stuck in her throat and choking her. Or she might end up with pneumonia from inhaling small bits.

What kind of quality of life would she be left with? Eating had been her one pleasure, at least until we'd begun to puree her food. I was gutlessly glad Yvonne, as the nurse, was the one to let Rebecca know about the stomach tube. Linda told me later that Rebecca had cried for the rest of the afternoon.

She stayed a day in the hospital for the procedure. A visiting nurse taught us how to use the funnel, how to clear the tube if it became blocked with the fibrous solution she got once a day, and what the feeding schedule should be. Rebecca hated it. She was cranky as soon as she returned from the hospital and had to submit to the feedings every four hours. We thought her bad mood had to do with the fact that she was out of control of yet another basic function of her life, which we understood and empathized with. But it turned out that some of the flavors tasted so bad to her that she would gag and even vomit within fifteen minutes of a feeding.

Faye was the first to catch on. One Sunday as she approached Rebecca with a can of vanilla-flavored supplement, Rebecca waved away the can, crying. Somehow Faye figured out the flavor was the problem. Even though the supplement was going down a tube and straight into her stomach, Rebecca could taste it, perhaps from belches or a bit of reflux. Faye made a note in the daily log, and the health-care staff launched an all-out effort to discover which flavors tasted best. Rebecca's top choice: butter pecan. They also figured out that a chaser of ginger ale helped with the flavors she liked least.

We tried to cheer her up. Residents tapped on her open door to say hello before leaving for appointments or programs, offering to wipe the saliva off her face or sit for a minute. Kimberly, the resident who had bonded most closely with her, bought Rebecca's scratch tickets every evening when she got her own. They sat together in front of the television, scratching away while one chatted and the other chortled. When the weather was nice, the interns wheeled her around the block or down to the Rite Aid. I got into the habit of popping in when she was watching her favorite, Maury Povich, whose guests almost always brawled, drawing spit-filled guffaws from Rebecca. At the start of parties, or when the women were crashing about the kitchen cooking, or when they had Comedy Central on in the TV room, someone usually remembered her and ran to her room to wheel her in.

Soon Jessie, who had moved in during November and was insecure about her position in the community, became envious of all the attention paid to Rebecca. She began complaining loudly in the dining room whenever staff was attending to Rebecca, who, volatile and impulsive in her anger with her increasingly circumscribed life, lashed out in her own way. That meant the right arm was wielded more frequently. It made for an extremely difficult situation, especially for the PCAs. The stage was set for another contentious staff meeting.

I floated an idea. "Can the interns pay more attention to Jessie? You know, read the newspaper with her, or walk her down to the CVS? Distract her when the PCAs are working with Rebecca."

"She just spoiled."

This was code for "You're spoiling Jessie, Carol," and it stung, but I held my tongue.

One of the PCAs thought Jessie didn't need more attention than she already got.

"Linda or me is up with her at four-thirty, three mornings a week, getting her ready for dialysis and fixing her breakfast. And we most always fix her dinner. She just don't like us paying attention to no one else."

"And Jessie can be kinda mean," Anna said. She was our AmeriCorps member, and she had a wonderful rapport with Rebecca that surely did not go unnoticed by Jessie. Not long after beginning her year at Miriam's House, Anna had created the communications book, with lovely artistry and an eye for bright color, from a five-by-seven photo album into which she put pages containing representations of elements of Rebecca's world: pictures taken from magazines, drawings of various staff member with their names underneath, words or phrases like *need changing* and *go outside*. Rebecca loved that little book to tatters. She kept it on her lap, referring to it as needed, laboriously turning the pages with her one good hand and pointing to the photo or the word that told us what she could not say for herself.

We talked about Rebecca's depression and how sensitive Jessie was. They were acting upset and frustrated, and who wouldn't be, I argued, unable to move from the chair or the bed or, like Jessie, stuck with dialysis three times a week? "I'd be a crazy woman if it were me."

The PCAs said that they understood all that but it was still hard trying to manage all the chores and medication distribution, cook for and take care of Rebecca, get Jessie to feel they hadn't forgotten her, and deal with all the other women as well. I tried reminding the PCAs about the many ways we had developed, over the years, to support and help them in these admittedly difficult jobs. Their pay was higher than that of almost all other PCAs in the city, even exceeding the living-wage standard. They had twenty annual leave days and liberal sick leave. A nurse was always on call, and they were never alone because Tim, the resident interns, and I were also in the house. They could speak up and work for change at every staff meeting.

Then I couldn't resist letting fly my version of a suck-it-up-and-do-your-jobs speech.

"This is why we're here, for these women, the Jessies and the Rebeccas, and not just women who pretty much take care of themselves. There's nowhere else for Jessie and Rebecca to go, let alone get the care and love they get here. It's our job, it's our mission to care for the ones labeled difficult." I stopped and looked around the circle, having to rather forcefully remind myself how dedicated they were, how much they cared. And I knew it was really hard work. But sometimes, tired of the complaints, I suspected they just wanted their jobs to be easier. Much like I wanted them to stop complaining and make my job easier.

We went back to the earlier plan. The interns would focus on Jessie, sitting at meals with her, taking her to Rite Aid, going outside with her while she smoked. And the PCAs would focus on Rebecca. If either of them became impossible, they could call me for intervention. So far, I had always been able to talk Jessie around, and Rebecca listened to both Yvonne and me.

Yvonne spoke in her deliberate, calm way. "I'll lecture Rebecca about her behavior. And let me know if she act up. Use the PCA log to make notes about it. I can always confront her again."

We all agreed to try the new plan. I was variously regarded as spoiling Jessie (an accusation that was to be repeated regularly over the next six years), not letting staff confront Rebecca hard enough, favoring staff over residents or residents over staff, and not understanding the work of PCAs because my job was admin, not frontline. I gritted my teeth, reminded myself I was not doing this work to win popularity contests, and tried to set my sights above my pettiness and staff's discontent.

The new system didn't go as smoothly as we hoped, of course. Everyone was compromising for the sake of the agreed-upon plan, which meant everyone felt unhappy with some aspect of it. PCAs wanted stricter consequences for Rebecca, interns felt Jessie was taking up too much time, and I just wanted everyone to shut up and do their jobs. Not that I ever said that. Not out loud.

Well, not out loud and in front of staff.

After a few weeks, the best Linda could say at staff meeting was, "I *guess* Rebecca be hitting at us less often."

We all laughed at Linda's expression, as dubious as her words. Jessie really was complaining less, and Rebecca really was trying to control her temper. It took some monitoring and a bit of intervention, but the two women were beginning to show some willingness to get along. Faye said she saw a difference on Sundays, and that the whole community felt different. "I even saw Jessie show Rebecca a page of her magazine, telling her about some murder."

Jessie and her murders. We smiled.

No longer frantic about her position in the community, Jessie either left Rebecca alone or made experimental attempts to reach out to her. Rebecca seemed to become accustomed to her stomach tube and began listening to Jessie's monologues about the murders in the newspaper and house gossip. Jessie loved the attention. Rebecca loved the communication. The two achieved a tentative peace.

We bumped along like this for several months until, early in 2003, Lawrice, the nurse we'd hired recently, told us about a consultation she'd had with the doctor about deterioration in Rebecca's strength. She could no longer pull herself onto her side for a diaper or clothing change, or help at all in the transfer from bed to wheelchair. The doctor decided Rebecca needed the higher level of care that a nursing home would give her. I called our licensing agency to ask if there were any way we could work it out for Rebecca to stay. They sent an inspector, who took one look at the stomach tube and told us we absolutely could not have someone so dependent in a community residence facility, and she should have been transferred as soon as the stomach tube had gone in.

We learned that Rebecca's physician was attending at a nursing home not far away in Northeast DC. They even had a couple of beds available. Though we hated the thought of Rebecca leaving us, this at least meant she'd be close enough for regular visits. We assumed we would only have to do the paperwork, move her in, and begin visiting. But a few days after our application was submitted, Yvonne came to my office with a strange expression on her face, telling me that the nursing home had rejected it. The manager told her Rebecca required too high a level of care, and they could not afford to give her a bed.

"I had to ask him twice to make sure I heard him. Makes no sense, how can you have too high a level of care for a nursing home? He said it again, so I came to talk to you."

"But that's what nursing homes *do*. I don't get it."

Chewing it over for the next five minutes didn't help either of us. We called him back on speaker phone and introduced ourselves. He began with the bald statement he'd already made to Yvonne: they'd rejected Rebecca's application because she needed too much care. We reminded him that her doctor, an attending at his nursing home, had herself recommended Rebecca. Again he said she needed too much attention, too much staff care.

Thankful he couldn't see our faces, on which expressions of incredulity and disgust mingled disrespectfully, we explained how little sense this made to us. What was a nursing home for if not to take care of a stroke victim who couldn't move or eat but was not ill enough to require hospitalization?

He said the care would be too expensive. That silenced us, mouths gaping at each other.

He tried again. "Her medications are too expensive. We can't afford her daily physical care plus the pharmacy expenses."

We ended the conversation and hung up the phone in disbelief. Then we got angry. Clearly she was being discriminated against as an AIDS patient. Yet we had to find a place for Rebecca, so we began looking at other DC nursing homes even as we fought to get her admitted at this one.

All of the DC nursing homes to which we applied rejected her application, whether or not they had beds available. I called a couple nurses I knew who had dealt with DC nursing homes and their policies for many years. What I learned, after promises were extracted from me not to quote them by name, gave me the answer but little comfort.

At that time, DC Medicaid paid providers like nursing homes one flat per diem rate per patient, regardless of the type or level of care they needed. Medications were reimbursed the same way. And so DC Medicaid reimbursed a nursing home resident who was fairly independent, needed minimal staff attention and relatively few medications at exactly the same dollar amount it reimbursed for a gravely ill, bed-bound patient with many and costly medications. The result was that nursing homes chose lower-level care patients over higher-level care patients in order to balance their budgets.

I hated the thought that DC nursing homes were cherry-picking residents, though as a business-owner myself I had to admit that I understood the need to operate in the red. But my sympathy ended there, because I also learned that the nursing homes fought any proposed change in Medicaid billing policies. Then I learned that Maryland had a three-tier reimbursement system in which higher levels of care were paid at higher rates and medication was reimbursed per expense, not on a flat per diem rate. We had often wondered why all the poorer DC residents we knew were staying in Maryland nursing homes. It turned out that, very simply, Maryland Medicaid had a better reimbursement policy.

Here was yet another item on the list of the often unseen discriminatory practices faced by our women.

The licensing agency was agitating for Rebecca's move and making threatening noises about our license. Finally we found a nursing home in Maryland, forty-five minutes away by car and two hours on public transportation. Nothing about this seemed right, especially that she had to go so far away, but we had no alternative. In a haze of misery, we prepared for her move.

***

Linda and I packed the van with everything going with Rebecca. It wasn't much. She was to have a bed in a four-person ward, and most of what was in her Miriam's House room had to be left behind or given to her daughter. We shut the van's back door and walked slowly to the house. Time to get Rebecca and go.

Yvonne had Rebecca ready, bundled against the February cold. Her head hung chin to chest, and she didn't look up or respond to us when we said, softly, that the van was ready. Yvonne went to the dining room to tell the gathered residents Rebecca was leaving. They followed along behind her, coming through the hallway door and gathering closely around Rebecca in her wheelchair. Still she did not lift her head. But the women tried.

"'Bye, Rebecca. I'll be missing you a lot.

"Don't you worry about nothing. Them folks there'll take real good care of you, and you can get better and come back here."

"Man, Becca, who I'm gonna scratch tickets with now?"

"Yvonne say you can come back for parties."

Rebecca shook her head.

"Don't cry, Rebecca. It'll be okay."

Finally we loaded the chair into the elevator. Linda got on with her and the rest of us waited for them in the entryway. We didn't talk. We held the front door open and they passed through, Linda pushing the wheelchair and telling Rebecca to put her scarf up, it's cold. We followed in a tight, still silent group under the cherry trees arching bare limbs toward an occluded sky. Linda helped Yvonne get Rebecca into the van. I climbed into the driver's side after heaving the wheelchair into the back. Linda sat down next to Rebecca, and Yvonne took the front passenger seat. As we pulled away from the curb, the little watching group waved, their hands describing small, shivery arcs in the frosty air.

The ride to the nursing home was long and very quiet. All I could hear was Rebecca's labored breathing and Linda's murmurs about wiping the spit off her coat. No one wanted the radio on. No one spoke. We drove far past the city of Silver Spring to an area I'd never visited. Finally I saw the place. As we pulled in, Rebecca began to sob.

We got out, shoulders hunched against the dreary day and its dreadful task, unloaded the few bags from the van, and settled Rebecca into her wheelchair. We found a ramped side entrance and entered the single-story brick building. Rebecca's sobs echoed, slapping the tiled floor and bare walls. We met with the social worker and the nurse, who took us to Rebecca's new room and indicated which of the four beds would be hers. Everything was neat and clean, but it wasn't Miriam's House, and still she cried.

While Yvonne and I went back to the admitting office to finalize details, Linda stayed with Rebecca to arrange her things. When we returned, the little bedside table was covered with a lacy cloth, and Rebecca's clothing was neatly placed in dresser drawers or hung up in the tiny closet shared with the woman in the next bed. A few photographs were taped to the wall. We said good-bye lovingly but quickly, not wanting to draw it out, bending over her hunched and shaking form for hugs that made contact but no impression. We left, Rebecca's

wordless lamentations pursuing us down the corridors and out
into the wretched day.

***

Round-trip visits to Rebecca took at least four hours, so I
couldn't go during business hours. The residents who were not
too ill to contemplate the trip were busy with appointments,
day programs, or GED classes. Linda spent one of her days off
with Rebecca, and Amanda, an intern, visited a couple days
later. They reported back that Rebecca had cried for at least
fifteen minutes, and they'd cheered her up with stories about
goings-on at Miriam's House. Someone said we should visit
more often, and a few of the residents and I decided to drive
out after dinner one evening. But when I called to make sure
we could visit at that time of day, the nurse told me Rebecca
was in the hospital. They had called for an ambulance just that
morning when her breathing had become alarmingly labored.

Kimberly, a couple other residents, and I drove to the hospital that evening, found Rebecca's room and tiptoed in. We
were quiet, not for fear of waking her up but because the figure
in the bed was thin and gray, so changed we had to look closely,
thinking we had come into the wrong room. We hadn't. It was
Rebecca. But she responded not at all: not to our voices, not
to our rubbing her hands, and not even to Kimberly holding
a scratch ticket under her nose, going at it frantically with a
dime and pleading in her gruff voice, "Ain't you wanna see if
you won?"

She was released from the hospital a few days later, only
to be readmitted within the week. Kimberly and I were on the
road once again on a frigid March evening, back at the hospital's front desk and asking for her room number, once more
entering a room and wondering if we'd made a mistake because

if anything, she was even thinner, grayer of face. Nor was she responsive. The nurse in the room with her when we arrived told me, as she left, that Rebecca was very, very ill.

But why? Why would she be so sick? When she'd left us just a few weeks before there had been no prognosis of imminent death, no talk of death at all. The move to the nursing home was supposed to help her, not make her worse. How could she be dying? How?

"Rebecca," I finally said, shaking away the questions and leaning over the bed to hold her hand. "Rebecca, it's me, it's Carol. Can you hear me? Kimberly's here, too."

No response.

Kimberly went around the bed and took Rebecca's other hand. "Becca! It's me and Miss Carol come to see you. Wake up, Becca, wake up. We here to see you."

No response.

"Becca!"

Feeling light-headed, I slumped into a chair. Kimberly bent over her friend, patting her head and calling, "Becca! *Becca!* Wake up!" I hadn't the heart to stop her. After a while a nurse came in, drawn, I guessed, by the shouts. She asked us to leave but didn't seem to mind when we were slow to do so and Kimberly was unable to hold back one last cry. "Wake up, Becca!"

We said nothing on the long drive home.

Two weeks later, the nursing home called me early one morning. Rebecca had died in her sleep the night before.

There was no funeral because her daughter spent the small grant we got for it on something else. Rebecca was buried in a pauper's grave somewhere near Baltimore, and we didn't know where. It was some consolation that we could have her memorial service as we always did for women who died, in the living room with the chairs and couches in a large circle, and the coffee table, covered in a purple shawl, in the middle. On it we placed the lit white pillar candle, tea lights, and the one-shoe-on, one-shoe-off photograph. One by one we got up to light a tea light from the pillar candle and tell Rebecca stories. We talked about how she loved to laugh, how much she could eat before the stomach tube went in, the way she listened to all the gossip, and wouldn't we want to know as much about her as she knew about us. The way she'd watch so intently when Kimberly scratched her lottery ticket. How much we missed her.

We tidied the room, pushing the couches back into place and stacking the chairs in the closet. We blew out the tea lights. Once more we admired the photo of Rebecca smiling and half-shod at Six Flags. I went to hang it back on the hallway wall as we scattered, knowing it would take a while to accustom ourselves to life without Rebecca.

I was about to put the photo on its nail when something caught my eye. I held it closer to get a better look at the glints of color showing up bright against the white shirt and one white sandal. It was crimson polish on her fingers and toes. I'd forgotten Linda had done her nails for the Six Flags trip. I stood there with the photo in my hand and imagined the two of them in Rebecca's room with a soap opera on the television and cotton pads and bottles of polish set out on the bedside table. Despite my sorrow, I smiled. But I also felt a stirring of the anger I'd held at bay in order to get myself and the community through the shock of her death. Her untimely death.

My hand trembled so much I missed the nail two times before getting that photo back in its place on the wall.

I filed a complaint at DC's Office of Human Rights against the DC nursing home that had refused to admit her. Some good had to come out of this mess, even if that might only be a reprimand or a demand to revise admission policies. Later I learned about the phenomenon called transfer trauma. Nursing-home staff are familiar with it: a new resident deteriorates and dies rather quickly, regardless of the level of health upon admission. The best explanation is the trauma, including depression and despair, of moving from home to institution.

For whatever reason, missed communication and/or the glacier-slow movement of the District of Columbia bureaucracy, I waited two summers for the city to act upon my human-rights complaint. Mary Ann Parker, attorney for the DC Long-Term Care Ombudsman Program at Legal Counsel for the Elderly, planned our strategy and accompanied me to the hearings. Thank God she did, for I was in over my head. Mary Ann, passionately committed to her work, was a formidable opponent, organized, intelligent, and calm. I sat by in awe.

The upshot of the complaint hearings was that they were required to add the word *AIDS* to the nondiscrimination clause in their admission policies. They never did admit why they'd denied Rebecca admission, which pissed me off. Nor that they were choosing residents at least partly based on what that admission would do to their bottom line.

The longer I worked at Miriam's House, the more I was forced to see the subtle and even outright discrimination perpetrated on our residents. No wonder they trusted so little. No wonder theirs was so often a worldview that allowed only for the implementation of an aggressive offense. The one assumption coming out of their life experience was that they had to fight for even the smallest crumb of respect, attention, or sustenance. Even my outrage was informative to me as I realized most of the residents were simply resigned to such circumstances in their own lives and those of the people around them.

Here is a fact: white, educated, middle- and upper-middle-class people like me cannot know what women like the residents of Miriam's House experience every day of their lives. We have no idea how it is to live one step from disaster in a world that shows, with no compunction, how little it cares. Yes, jobs and savings can be lost, but we will never lose our education, health from a lifetime of good medical care and proper nutrition, and safety nets in the form of support systems or a relatively well-off family. We may lose wealth, but there's a big difference between becoming poorer and living in poverty.

Furthermore, our emotions are a by-product of our privilege. Some of us shrug our shoulders and turn away, grousing about lazy people, welfare queens, immoral behavior, and the breakdown of the family, unwilling to admit that the happenstance of birth, not our own worthiness, placed us in a position that made prosperity, industry, and even morality possible. My outrage, itself, was indicative of an easier life. I had never been treated the way these women had always been treated, nor, until my move to DC, had I known anyone who had. I had the energy to be angry because cruelty, poverty, and neglect had not beaten all inspiration out of me. That is not to say that residents and staff were not upset or angry in their own way. But the contrast in amount and level between my emotions and theirs was striking to me.

Living, Rebecca showed me what grace was, as she participated in life despite her terrible limitations. Dying, she made me see the pervasive and profound disenfranchisement that results from America's offhanded treatment of its vulnerable ones. Dead, she helped me to understand that my blessings blind me even as I try to see. Hers was no success story, nothing to brag about to people asking us about program outcomes and resident triumphs.

Rebecca's was only a story about courage and sheer stamina to live valiantly the life that imprisoned her.

CHAPTER TWENTY-FOUR

In February 2002 residents began reporting seeing Gina, whom I had moved to her uncle's house the previous December, at the hospital or clinic. They said she didn't look good, and she wanted to come back. I had to restrain my impulse to jump into the van and go get her (What if she looked bad because she was using? What about my own values around collective decision-making?). I brought the subject up in the next team meeting, trying not to sound as eager as I was. We agreed that Yvonne would call Gina's uncle to find out more about her health.

Her uncle reported that Gina had begun declining just after the new year. She had been admitted twice recently to the hospital for weeklong stays. She was weaker, sleeping a lot, and physically debilitated by kidney dialysis three days a week. Yvonne and I agreed that the situation warranted polling staff about Gina's return. So we brought it up at the next Thursday meeting. To my joy, all agreed that Gina should return to us. The PCAs, who would be the most affected by her return because she was ill and would need a lot of care from them, were also the most outspoken in favor of letting her return.

"She need to come back. She ain't getting the care she need at her uncle's, not that he ain't love her, but he can't help her like we can."

"I've been missing Gina anyway. I'd like her back here."

"She can have her old room. I'll fix it up for her. And it sounds like you should order a hospital bed for her, Yvonne."

"Yeah, but first let's see if Medicaid says so."

"Ain't no one love her like we do. I bet she come back and get better right away."

We called a special house meeting the next day, hopeful but unsure about what the women would say. They'd been so adamant about her leaving. Yvonne opened the meeting by explaining the reason we had called it. She described, without breaking confidentiality, something of what Gina was going through. I acknowledged the reality about how Gina had left us. We then laid out the reasons for staff's willingness to bring her home. We told them they were important in this discussion and we needed to hear from them, no matter what they had to say. And then, we waited.

The women shifted in their chairs, looking sideways at one another and then down at their feet. I concentrated on keeping my face neutral. Kimberly spoke up first.

"Miriam's House gave me a second chance, hell, a third chance even. I think we gotta give Gina another chance, too."

"I seen her. She look awful, she need us right now."

"She know she did wrong. She ain't gonna do it again."

"She need some of Elsie's care and them Sunday dinners cooked by Faye. Then she'll be better."

"She ain't using. And she feel real bad about bringing that beer for Terri."

And so within a week, grinning like a fool, I was driving out to Silver Spring. I had no sooner pulled in front of the house and stepped out of the van than Gina was coming out the front door as fast as she could, feebly but with that crooked smile on her face and a bag in her hand. We grabbed each other in an ecstatic hug. She threw the bag into the van, hollered another good-bye to her uncle standing at the door, and got in.

"Take me home."

She then criticized the route I took, directing me on what she was sure was a shortcut while poking at me for not knowing it already. And who cared? She was coming home.

**

I was on duty one evening about a week later when Gina's difficulties breathing made us call 911. I followed on foot to Howard Hospital, only a few blocks away, and went inside to find her on a stretcher in the hall because there were no bays available. We settled in for what became a long and chaotic wait that did have two redeeming features—Gina spouted endless and hilarious commentary, and a drunk patient obligingly provided her with something on which to remark. Gina first noticed him when something moved on what had looked like an empty stretcher parked in a nearby corner.

"It's alive!" Gina might have imagined her whisper actually was a whisper. She would have been deluding herself.

"Good Lord, Gina, you scared me." I noticed out of the corner of my eye that I was not the only one.

"Here we go again. Why do weird shit always happen when you bring me to the ER?" She was speaking to me but keeping a cautious eye on the stretcher. Since I was on her right and the stretcher was to her left, her head was turned away from me. This meant that she had to ditch entirely the effort to whisper in favor of her normal tone of voice, always impressive in its ability to cut through ambient noise.

"I could say the same thing to you."

"What*e*ver. Did you see that thing move?"

She was staring at the stretcher, and though I had not noticed movement, I watched it for a moment. It looked like a pile of dirty sheets plunked down haphazardly, ready for laundry services. Suddenly, as if on cue, an arm fell out from under the disorderly pile.

Gina jumped. "Shit!"

I had jumped, too, along with the others around us now forming what could only be termed an audience.

"See? See? It's alive!"

"Could you watch your language? Others can hear you."

Some small part of me realized I sounded prissy, but I couldn't stop myself and was well aware of Gina's potential for flamboyant and dramatic scenes. Hopefully she would not notice the amused and interested expressions on the faces around her. That would be all she needed.

She was paying me no mind, going on about the guy about to fall off his stretcher and I should go catch him. *Fat chance,* I thought, as she let loose another *shit.*

"Would you hush? He's drunk. Not someone I want to tangle with right now."

Gina snorted in amusement, picturing, I assumed, me in a struggle for control over this rather large, certainly drunk man as he half climbed, half fell from the stretcher. She had no time to share her imaginings, however, because he staggered a few steps forward as though about to fall flat.

"Watch out!" Gina's call was far more disquieting than the poor man's stumble and had a far more startling effect on those within earshot, which, given the piercing nature of her voice, was essentially the entire ER. "He falling!"

Drawn by her stentorian tones, ER personnel rushed over. After a brief struggle, the guards succeeded in getting him to lean against the wall, support that seemed to please him in a way that the idea of lying down again had not. Apparently believing their help was no longer needed, the security guards walked back to their station. Soon, and with the slow deliberation of the alcohol-impaired mind, the man began to unbutton his shirt.

Gina made a disgusted face but did not turn from her avid watching. "Ain't had a shower in forever, I bet. Yuck."

At this stage I had dropped all pretense and was staring as much as anyone. I didn't add color commentary, but then, it wasn't needed. Gina was all over it. "That nasty shirt, who wears a shirt like that? If something crawl out of it, I'ma pitch a fit. Nasty thing."

But not even Gina was equal to the task of maintaining running chatter when, swaying on his feet, our drunken entertainer began to fumble with his zipper. Mouth agape, she watched as he unzipped his pants. "Oooooooh, lord."

With the settling of his pants around his ankles came the realization he wore no undergarment.

Gina dug a sharp elbow into my arm. "I see it! I see it!"

Another dig. "Carol, do you see it?"

Just about then the security guards rushed back and hustled the poor man toward the bathroom. Gina dug again, elbow to my forearm, asking her question. Clearly she was not going to shut up unless she got her response. I sighed. "Yes, Gina, I saw it."

Naturally, my admission amused Gina exceedingly, her amusement lasting through the evening and well past our return to Miriam's House the next morning. Gina got a lot of mileage out of the story of the drunk guy dropping his drawers

right in front of Carol, almost all of which I heard about secondhand from highly amused staff members.

**

The kitchen at Miriam's House got really hot in the
summertime. Appliance motors on the ice machine, the three-
door refrigerator, a freezer, a ten-burner stove, and two ovens
kicked out enough heat to fill even this fairly large space. Several
ceiling vents releasing an air-conditioned breeze couldn't keep
up. So on the Sunday after our ER adventure, making breakfast
in that hot kitchen and with a migraine coming on, I was
struggling to maintain my composure.

"Hey, whatcha cooking?" Gina, recently out of bed, judging
from the state of her hair.

"Pancakes, bacon, home fries . . ."

She didn't let me finish the list. "Blueberry pancakes?"

I eyed her warily. "Well, no, Gina, not this week."

Uh oh.

"You know that's my favorite. Last time you made them
you ain't even made your blueberry syrup to go with 'em." Gina
never exactly pouted, but I had never known anyone who could
so effortlessly assume an air of bruised betrayal. I avoided looking at her face, aware that my control over my temper was at
gossamer strength. The bacon needed tending, so I masked my
unwillingness to look Gina in the eyes by bustling with great
concern over to the electric frying pan, spatula at the ready.
Without looking up, I spoke again.

"Blueberries are out of season. And not all the residents
like them, so I thought plain would be a good change."

She muttered something about frozen berries. "And anyway, you said you'd make blueberry, remember? At the ER?
When that guy took off his pants in front of you?"

"Good grief, Gina, it wasn't in front of *me*, really, and how do you expect me to . . ." Suddenly, the five or six women waiting in the dining room rushed in. They had overheard the phrase *took off his pants in front of you*.

"What? What?"

"Took his pants off in front of Miss Carol? When?"

"Naked? With Carol right there?"

Eager interest in this juicy story made them deaf to my pleas to get out of the hot, now crowded kitchen. Gina, inveterate lover of attention, was in her element. "Falls right off his stretcher thing in the ER and stumbles around, like he ain't know where he is. Drunk and . . ."

"Get out of the kitchen! How am I supposed to cook?"

As I rarely lost my temper, at least, not in front of the residents, six chastened women left in rather a hurry, surprised, I should guess, by my vehemence. Immediately, I felt guilty for shouting at them. I turned my frayed attention back to the bacon. The burning bacon. Time for a deep breath, a sip of tea, a gathering of the shredded remnants of my patience. Gina and her audience were huddled at a dining table for the highly dramatized, I had no doubt, denouement of the story. Great. Plain pancakes and burned bacon for breakfast and I'm hot and my head is getting worse.

At that moment, Gina's voice rose above its stage whisper. I could hear her from my position by the stove and recognized in her tone the approaching high point of the story. A happily horrified gasp came from the women clustered around Gina as she produced the coup de grace:

"We saw it."

***

I have so often wished that we had known Laila before she came to Miriam's House in March 2002. Lawrice, our nurse at the time, was passionate about getting Laila admitted. I was acting as program director because we were between hires, which meant I became more involved with this intake than was usual for me. After Lawrice's first visit to meet Laila's case manager, she came to me to advocate for Laila's admittance. There were some obstacles in the way, and although that in itself was not unusual, Lawrice was committed to making sure we dealt with all of them successfully.

The National Institutes of Health (NIH), whose hospital had a wonderful HIV/AIDS department, referred Laila to us. We'd had several referrals from NIH over the years, and there was great mutual respect between our two organizations. Our residents received absolutely the best treatment there.

The best, in this case, also meant some convenience for Miriam's House. Most practically, we didn't have to worry about transport all the way out Connecticut Avenue to Rockville, Maryland—a trip that could take forty-five minutes one way, depending on traffic—because NIH provided transportation there and back. The staff time saved was most helpful. With wonderful, individualized care and the most up-to-date methods, medicine, and equipment, we almost always found that the women treated there improved in health. The one sad exception was Laila, who, by the time she got to us, was so sick that she spent more days in the hospital than she did at Miriam's House.

When Laila was just a girl, living in her native Africa, she was injured in a car accident and bled so much she required a blood transfusion. Her mother, a nurse, signed the papers that allowed for the transfusion and other treatments. That decision seemed so obvious at the time: of course, if my little girl needs blood, then give it to her. Without any other thought than that, she had signed.

Within a couple of years, when she was thirteen, Laila began suffering strange maladies and infections. A doctor noticed in her records the blood transfusion of two years before and suggested an HIV test. Though horrified at the mere possibility, Laila's mother agreed. When the test returned positive, she became overwhelmed with sorrow and guilt. She began searching throughout Africa for the best medical care and the best doctors. Staying busy planning, phoning, and traveling on behalf of her precious daughter helped to hold at bay an ever-present thought: my daughter has AIDS because of a decision I made.

Inevitably, Laila's condition deteriorated because the available medical care was spotty and not necessarily modern. It became clear that if she wanted her daughter to have any chance at life, she would have to consider sending her to live with relatives in the States. It was a stark choice. She could keep Laila home and comfortable through her last months, or send her half a world away for the best medical care and the possibility of recovery.

She sent her daughter to the States.

I learned this story in part from the case manager at NIH who referred Laila to Miriam's House. The rest I learned from Laila's mother herself, when she sat for an hour one day in my office during one of her few visits, weeping for her daughter, the transfusion that infected her, and her part in the misery. I met her only this one time. She was unable to make the long trip very often because her travel visa strictly limited the number and length of trips to the States, and she had Laila's brothers and sisters at home. This visit turned out to be the last one during which she could see her daughter alive. The next trip, only a few months later in July, was for Laila's funeral.

We learned something else from the NIH case manager, something I think Laila's mother never knew. Laila's American relatives, terrified of AIDS, had isolated her in a room apart, feeding her on paper plates with plastic utensils, keeping her away from everyone else living there, rarely allowing her out for family gatherings or functions at the high school she attended.

So by the time she arrived at Miriam's House, Laila was not only very ill but she rarely smiled and hardly wanted to come out of her room, though we encouraged her to. She spoke in a high, whispery voice, usually to complain in a tone I could only think of as resembling most strongly the whining of a ten-year-old. When I would go to her room to check on her, she was usually in bed with the covers over her head. We had trouble getting her to eat and couldn't persuade her to come down-stairs to our celebrations. She didn't go out except when NIH transport came for her.

Thank God for NIH. Not only did they give Laila compassionate care that must have seemed a lifeline to her, they had also enrolled her in the one redeeming and shining light in the final stage of her life: Camp Heartland in California. If Laila ever smiled, it was when talking about her camp experiences, all the friends she had there, and how much the staff loved her. We had direct confirmation of this when NIH helped us contact Camp Heartland so I could tell staff members about Laila's failing health and thank them for what they had meant to her. During the call, I asked them about Laila at camp.

The Laila they knew was vivacious, friendly with everyone she met, kind to the younger children, popular with all of her peers, and always up for adventures like playing harmless practical jokes on staff. They spoke of a young woman of vibrant energy, talent, and a wonderful sense of fun, a person of whom we at Miriam's House had seen only the feeblest glimmer.

One of the reasons I'd called Camp Heartland that day was to tell them she was not expected to live much longer. They promised to inform Laila's friends for us, a special one in particular whom they wouldn't name. They did, however, hold out the possibility of a visit from this person, possibly on her birthday in a few weeks.

***

On Laila's birthday, Lawrice and I drove out Connecticut Avenue to the NIH campus. Lawrice told me that Laila had been unable to speak on the phone when Lawrice had called her the day before. We didn't talk any more until we'd parked the car and were in the hospital. We stopped at the nurses' station to check in with Laila's nurse, and someone asked if we wanted to go to the birthday party. They had cake in the meeting room, and the special guest had come from California. We said we'd come later, after spending time with Laila.

Laila's room was a single, dark because the light was off and the window blind down. Her bed occupied a space mid-room against the far wall. We couldn't tell if she was asleep or unconscious even though the nurse had told us earlier in the morning that Laila had seemed to understand the reason for the cake. She'd recognized the friend just arrived from California and had been joyful, to the extent that a dying teenager can be, at seeing him.

From either side of the bed we each took up a cold hand and tried to warm it between ours. We watched her face for a sign of consciousness. We softly called her name and did not cease for some time, even though we could see she was not aware. Yet we stayed, unwilling to admit by any word or chance movement the pressing weight of helplessness.

One of the nurses appeared at the door, motioning to us. We left Laila's side.

"Have you met Chris?"

Her excitement grated. She smiled and we experienced a moment of disorientation. But he had come all the way from California, this friend, this Chris, and the nurse was strangely insistent that we should meet him. We could thank him, she said, and maybe tell him something about Laila. She led us eagerly down the hall to the meeting room. We followed, lagging behind, still seeing Laila in that bed. And then, there was the cake on the table in the center of the room, the *Happy Birthday* banner on the wall, and colorful paper plates and napkins. Balloons. There were the people sitting in chairs that lined the perimeter of the room. Here in this room down the hall from where Laila was dying.

"Chris, this is the director and nurse from Miriam's House, where Laila has been living."

A slim black man unfolded long limbs to stand before us and look at us with beautiful, large eyes that probably usually laughed but today looked weary, and I thought about how he had come to visit his friend who was dying so young.

"Carol and Lawrice, this is Chris Tucker."

The comedian reached out a slender, long hand. He said hello and I thought he seemed shy, or maybe he was tired of all the starstruck people pressing around him. We shook his hand. None of us spoke.

Laila's funeral was lovely and the July day on which it was held, sunny and crisp. Brightly handsome young people stood at the doors and in the aisles. They handed a single long-stem yellow rose, Laila's favorite flower, to each one of us.

***

No matter how much a death affected me, there was always the community to love and the business that needed attention. There were always the women, each in her own way making Miriam's House a home, each in her own way coping with her life, illness, and sobriety. It always made for an interesting mix, one that often brought together the sublime and the ridiculous.

While she was with us, it was often Terri representing the ridiculous side.

***

Terri was uncomfortable. With her gregarious personality, this meant that the whole house knew she was uncomfortable, why, and exactly what the doctor had told her to do about it. This wouldn't be remarkable—after all, the house was filled with women living with AIDS and various other health and physical disabilities—except that Terri had no discretion when it came to what might be considered a delicate subject. Well, what I considered a delicate subject.

Terri had genital warts and herpes. Both.

"Miss Carol, I be a mess down there. Can't hardly sit still."

I had just entered the dining room on some errand, and there was Terri, pacing restlessly.

"Um. Oh." Given as many conversations as I'd had about women and their health, one might think I could come up with something more articulate, or at least sympathetic.

"Seriously, you should see it. Doctor said he ain't never seen nothing like it. Can't sit, can't walk, can't lie down without it hurting."

"Terri, do the nurses know about this? You should tell them." I always tried to be a good listener even while guiding residents to the appropriate staff, so I did attempt not to emphasize the word *them* too much. That I backed away even as I de-emphasized may have negated the effort. Terri forced me to admit to my prim-and-proper side. Inherited from Victorian ancestors, no doubt.

A night or two later, as I was doing the final walk-through after my duty shift, I heard voices when I passed Terri's door. Wanting to check in, I knocked and entered. Linda, the PCA on shift, stood just inside the doorway. Later, I recalled the odd look in her eyes when she glanced at me as I came in. That look and her position barely inside the room instead of near Terri on her bed might have clued me in, had I paid attention.

"Hey, Terri, how come you're not asleep? It's late."

I'd asked for it.

"Because," she told me, "these damned warts ain't let me sleep. It's like I got something between my legs, like a balloon, real uncomfortable. Got a mirror and looked at it, but now I wish I hadn't. It look like a catcher's mitt down there, all swolled up."

"So, you were letting Linda know? So Linda can call the nurses?" Once again I backed away from Terri, coldheartedly ignoring Linda's desperate glance as I prepared my exit. I liked to think of myself as a compassionate person, but I had my limits.

"Nurses can't do nothing. I just gotta wait for the medicine to work, that's what the doctor said."

"She just took the night dose." Linda's shifting feet moved her no closer to Terri. "But you need to take this stuff for a few days to notice any difference."

I muttered something like oh, all right then, well, okay, um, I should finish my walk-through, um, so I'll just . . . when Terri interrupted me, sitting up in bed and throwing back the sheet.

"Like a damn catcher's mitt. You should see it."

"No!" Linda and I were uniformly adamant.

"Don't you believe me? It's true, look." She began to draw her feet out from under the sheet.

In her haste to get out, Linda plainly forgot my presence just behind her, holding the door halfway open but also blocking it. And I was similarly on the move. Our common impulse to flee caused her to back up, stumbling over my right foot. It caused me to step quickly into the hallway with the door beginning to close. Linda, loathe to be left in that room, grabbed the inner door handle and yanked. I, opposed to being drawn into that room, grabbed the outer door handle and yanked. Simultaneously I tried to untangle my right leg from hers so that it could join my left leg out in the hallway, a need that competed with Linda's unwillingness to move *her* leg because that would have meant stepping back into the room toward Terri, who was preparing to display her . . . condition.

All we wanted was to get ourselves on the right side of the door. The hallway side. This single-minded desire, held rather strongly by both of us, overtook our attempts to disentangle our legs, so that we simply tumbled out of the room in undignified haste, looking, I'm sure, like a pair of Keystone Kops. Who never had Terri to contend with.

I dreaded seeing Terri the next day, certain she would feel hurt at my abandonment. She came through the kitchen hallway door just as I was trying to slip unnoticed into my office.

"Hey, Miss Caroll Just met with Yvonne. She say I should feel better in a couple of days."

She didn't seem upset with me, but I looked at her cautiously and murmured that I was happy to hear the good news. With some show of energetic purpose I put my key into the lock. But Terri was never one to take a hint, and she was not done with me. She wondered aloud if she'd ever look, you know, normal. You know, down there.

Again, I referred her to Yvonne.

She deflected my suggestion, launching heartlessly into a story about how, when she was out there living the life, you know, she had met up with some guy behind the Sunoco for "well, you know. So we go behind the building and get started . . ."

Oh, good lord.

"No, wait, this is funny. So he puts his hand down there. Jumps back, throws the packet at me, and runs away." She giggled. "Scared the shit out of him so bad he gave me the hit for free."

Just then I had to hastily excuse myself because my telephone began to ring.

Really, it did.

CHAPTER TWENTY-FIVE

You couldn't look at Jessie and not make immediate and uncomplimentary assumptions about her intellectual abilities. Her left eye looked out at the world at an upward forty-five-degree angle. The effect, quite strange in and of itself, was made the more so because hers were large eyes, set rather far apart in her very round face. Had her eyes not been so afflicted, they would have been strikingly beautiful, as they were on the faces of each of her four daughters. As it was, one was rarely certain about which eye to look at nor able to determine whether she was directing her conversation to a particular person or to the room in general.

Jessie was short, round of torso, with very bowed legs. A long, white scar slashed across her face, above a similar one on her neck underneath her left ear. What hair she did possess was either plastered onto her scalp with hair grease or allowed to spring up in a fuzzy fringe. She dressed as though she'd grabbed the first garments that came to hand in the morning, with no reference whatsoever to a mirror, fashion convention, or color coordination.

I adored her. I also spent a good bit of time chasing after her because she seemed to listen better to me than to anyone else and because Jessie required a good deal of chasing. She once got out of her bed in a Southeast DC hospital, put on her clothes, left the room, and walked out the front door without saying anything to anyone, leaving me to discover her absence when I went to visit her one afternoon. The panic—mine and the hospital's—lasted an hour, until Donna called me from Miriam's House to say Jessie was out front demanding that someone pay the taxi driver for her.

We'd already discovered during Rebecca's sojourn with us how jealous Jessie could be of attention paid to other residents. But she had a certain charm and could get along well when she cared to. She would sit with Gina in the dining room, reading up about recent murders and relaying the gory details to anyone who came into the room. Jessie and Kimberly were best friends when they weren't fighting like pissed-off alley cats. And how Jessie loved her crabs! Early in the warmer months when she still had money, she'd buy half a bushel, spread newspaper out over a dining-room table, and feast for an entire afternoon.

I was glad Jessie and Gina got along. It could have been an explosive mix, both of them needy of attention yet convinced they weren't worthy of it. But Gina was not well at all. As it turned out, I had little enough time left to worry about her.

***

One Saturday afternoon in November 2002, we made an emergency call for Gina when she collapsed in the hallway near the front office, barely breathing. In the flurry of activity—me making the 911 call, Elsie putting together the paperwork to send with her, and anxious women standing about—*You'll be okay, Gina*—we had no thought that this might actually be the last time for such tumult around Gina. It seemed like one more ER trip among many. So I walked the four blocks to Howard Hospital and sat in the emergency-room waiting area with nothing more on my mind than relief I'd remembered to bring a bottle of water and a magazine.

It didn't occur to me to worry when the charge nurse wouldn't let me sit with Gina in the treatment area, something rare at Howard Hospital ER back then. Nor would she tell me anything except that the doctors were with Gina. Finally, someone came out to tell me that Gina was being transferred to a room. To my horror, I recognized the floor and wing as the intensive-care unit (ICU).

I stopped long enough to call Tim, then took the elevator up to the ICU and asked to see Gina, but was told I couldn't just then as the doctors were with her and she was being intubated. I was directed to the ICU waiting room, a cheerless, chilly room already familiar from other interminable-seeming waits. After a long time and two calls to keep Tim and Elsie informed, I was allowed into the ICU bay, where the ventilator hissed rhythmically to the up-and-down of Gina's chest.

I have sat waiting for death at many an ICU bedside, with its technological marvels and lifesaving machines all holding out the dwindling hope that the end might never come. And I have sat waiting for death in many a woman's bedroom with nothing but the comfort of clean sheets and cool washcloths, pain medications, and hands that massage sweet-smelling lotion onto dry skin, all with no hope except to make the dying as comfortable as possible. For myself I would choose the latter.

Yet I didn't get to choose for anyone else, and what Gina wanted was all-out effort to save her life, no matter what. As a result, we—Tim, the residents, staff, and I—would wait by her bed as machines forced air into her lungs and the life seeped out of her invaded body. Our one consolation was this: we were honoring Gina's choice.

After I saw Gina, the ICU staff allowed me to use the desk phone to call Tim and Elsie. I told them about Gina and asked Tim to call her uncle, then help Elsie tell the women. I said I'd wait for anyone who wanted to come to the hospital, and he offered to drive a group up in the van. Then, sick of breathing the moribund air, I wandered outside around the plaza that fronted on Georgia Avenue, letting the breeze wash away the ICU smells in my nostrils, clothing, and hair. It was only four o'clock and beginning to get dark on a crisp November day, unusual weather for humid Washington, DC. As I paced, I pictured the group of them together listening to Tim and Elsie. I could picture it because we'd called such meetings so many times.

They would gather quickly, apprehensively, in the dining room. Rarely was it good news when one of these sudden meetings was called. Anyway, they would have seen the expressions on Tim's and Elsie's faces, who would wait until everyone was there before they explained that Gina was on a ventilator at Howard Hospital, unconscious.

After a flurry of questions and exclamations, the women would swirl away to get ready to leave or set about making their meal so they could visit later. A couple residents would decide not to go and would sit quietly while the rest headed purposefully away to kitchen or bedroom. Of those, one would grab a Bible, trying to remember Gina's favorite verses. Another would remind herself to bring an extra sweater because the ICU always seemed so cold. Two would agree to go in to see Gina together because they wanted to pray over her. The others would be whirling about the kitchen, making their evening meal quickly in order to be ready in time for Tim's return with the first group. The ones who couldn't stand to see their friend in such a state would try to assuage their guilt by sending complicated messages that no one would remember to relay because the sight of Gina in that bed with that machine living her life for her would strike all thoughts from the heads of the message-bearers.

They poured into the waiting room in a cloak of fresh air, asking if I was all right and had I seen Val. I described what they'd find in that ICU bay, hoping to mitigate the shock. I sat and waited as the women, two by two, visited. No one was gone very long, and they returned quietly, some of them avoiding looking at the rest of us as they flung themselves into chairs, some pacing and wishing aloud to go home.

Tim drove that first group back, returned in half an hour with the second group, and we repeated the process. After they left and I'd clasped Gina's hand once again—*I'll make blueberry pancakes for you, and syrup, too. I promise*—and Tim had driven off in the van, I walked home, needing time to be alone, reflect, and let what had happened sink in.

The next day, Sunday, Tim and I walked back to the hospital. Gina's family had not yet arrived, so we had her to ourselves for a while. The room was cramped. The hospital's character-istic smells intensified in the cramped space, as did the heavy-hanging air of morbidity. When an ICU nurse bustled in to manage Gina's care and monitor the workings of the machines, it was almost a relief. At least she was human. ICU nurses always suspended the two-person-only rule and let us stay en masse when a woman was dying. The room, already crowded with its poles and tubes and machines and power cords snak-ing along the floor, was made more so by our group hovering around the bed. I knew we were making their work that much more difficult. But they always gave us those final moments.

By the time the five or six members of her family had arrived, Gina was failing, and we were not asked to keep the two-visitors rule. Tim and I explained what we knew to her family. We fell silent.

What to do when death is on its way? The default decision in an ICU room is to stare at the monitors displaying vital signs because, I think, there is some anchoring familiarity in a screen with information on it. The hypnotic effect of the changing numbers and steady hiss from the ventilator rivet people's attention as though by the very force of concentration they can forestall what's coming.

Realizing Gina's family was mesmerized in this way, yet unwilling to allow hissing and beeping be the last things she heard, I stepped forward to lean over my dying friend and hold her cold hand in mine.

"I love you, Gina. We all love you."

Tim joined me, his hand over mine over Gina's. Speechless, I could only look at her family as we backed away from her side.

Reading my expression, her uncle hastened forward. The others in the room took his cue, gathering around her bed several moments before the lines flattened and the measured beeping became a single unending tone.

Good-bye, Gina. We love you.

CHAPTER TWENTY-SIX

As winter turned slowly to spring in 2003, the women played hard-fought bingo, sharing some of the prizes they'd won with our newest resident, Denise, who had been admitted under hospice care and was too ill to play. We celebrated our seventh anniversary with the usual traditions: piles of homemade food cooked by residents and staff, a program led by a resident and board member paired as emcees, Yvonne reading a poem she'd written for the occasion, and our traditional ritual that included saying the names of the women who had died and lighting tea candles for each. Jackee, a recently admitted resident, sang a song that she mercifully cut a lot shorter than her typical serenades, much to our collective relief. We missed Rebecca, some staff members grieving long into the summer. And the house had lost a bit of its brightness with Gina gone.

Tim, a couple of the board members, some staff and I were busy with an application for the annual Washington Post Award for Excellence in Nonprofit Management. There were three rounds for weeding out candidates until a final five would be announced in May. Our initial goal was to make it to the second round. When we were told in January we'd passed the first cut, we felt like the rest of the process was icing on the cake. We commenced work on the imposing second round with its long list of questions requiring detailed answers. We would set up in the staff lounge on the ground floor or in the rec room if we wanted more space. There, around a table, board members and staff worked together to answer the questions, proof the most recent draft, and eat pizza. In the bright light and loud congeniality of those meetings we talked about Miriam's House, its strengths and weaknesses, its successes and mistakes, all of us together, laughing, interrupting one another, giggling at the way my writing was sometimes burdened with unnecessary detail (*the large, heavy green notebook*), while chomping on pizza and brownies.

After one such meeting, I stood outside on the front walkway, saying good-bye and thank you to board members and staff. Their voices faded into the chill night, car motors revved and headlights blinked on. For a moment I stood alone, breathing deeply the moist air, its cool touch soothing after the boisterous activity in the rec room's heat. As I began to relax, a thought released from where I'd been keeping it submerged these hours: Denise was dying.

Elsie heard people leaving. She came out the front door to stand quietly beside me and tell me Denise's condition had not changed during the time I was in the meeting. She and Megan, one of the resident interns, had bathed her. They'd combed her scant hair and dressed her in a clean gown and massaged lotion into skin hanging loosely on withered limbs.

And we stood there at the far margin of light streaming from the glass-paneled door, so close to the night that we cast no shadow, suspended, attentive for this moment to what was between. Then, without speaking, we turned back to Miriam's House.

Denise's room was tidy, dark, peaceful, the familiar wheeled cart placed against a wall, a single chair next to her bed. I sat down. She was barely visible in the gloom. She breathed quietly, evenly, eyes closed, motionless save for the slight, very slight, rise and fall of the sheet folded neatly over her chest. I gazed at her face, mercilessly reduced by wasting's whittling hand, all sharp nose and cheekbone and chin. We were still, she and I. We were still in that room, in the curtained dark, held in thrall at the borderland.

***

Denise died a few days later. Jessie went back into the hospital with a high fever of unknown cause. When I visited her at Washington Hospital Center, she talked incessantly about Denise, how she had sat with her the night before she died; how a few weeks earlier she'd found Denise on the floor, gripped by a violent seizure, and alerted Yvonne; how sad she was her friend was gone yet how glad that Denise had died at Miriam's House. "I ain't never want to go anywhere else, Miss Carol. I'll be staying forever."

A resident celebrated her seventh sobriety anniversary. Tim carried the grill out to the patio in late April, and Faye began to grill Sunday dinners. Jessie's daughter had a second baby. Early in May we were told that Miriam's House had been chosen as one of five finalists for the award, so we prepared for the final round—a site visit from the committee. Young male relatives of two residents were shot and killed on the streets of DC. Another resident attended the trial of the man who had killed her daughter two years before, and when he was sentenced to forty-four years she came home fiercely, tearfully exultant. Amanda, the intern especially beloved of Jessie, took the residents to the annual Kite Festival on the national mall, and out in the van to take advantage of Free Scoop Night at the Ben and Jerry's in Adams Morgan. Stephanie, AmeriCorps member, reported that Jessie and Chloe were sitting on our front patio when Chloe vomited all over the bricks, having not made it in time to the grass. Jessie, watching her and already tender of stomach herself, vomited empathetically right where she sat, splattering her shoes, the table and chair legs, and making Chloe laugh. The two of them were so tickled by the event they were helpless to aid with the cleanup, according to Stephanie, laughing so hard they couldn't do anything but shout about how it had been the funniest thing *ever* while Stephanie brought out bucket after bucket of hot, soapy water.

I watched the daytime Emmys with Jessie, who knew every actor and which show they were on, jumping up and down at announcements of the winners, extravagantly pleased for them all. I sat in pleasant companionship with Kimberly one evening watching a gospel-music awards show, but broke the mood with a sharply critical comment about a female duo that, to me, looked more like they were dressed and performing for a Las Vegas act than for a gospel concert. "How is that about Jesus?" I grumbled intemperately, but then sat red-faced when Kimberly retorted, "Ain't everyone got to worship the way you worship, Carol." All I could do was say "You're right and I'm sorry, Kimberly," and we were silent for a while until Kimberly took up once more what I had interrupted, singing along with the acts, clapping her hands and chair-dancing.

Terri called in from the front door after her curfew one evening in late May. There she stood, looking pathetic, when I stepped out to confront her about being late. As I steered her toward a patio chair, she began a voluble outburst.

"I ain't used, Miss Carol," she said as we sat down. "I swear. I ain't used, I be late cuz of the bus." She embarked on a long and detailed explanation of how that damn bus had thwarted her earnest attempts to make curfew, stating with bug-eyed vehemence that she had not used. "I swear, I ain't used this time, I swear on my mother's grave."

Terri's mother was alive and well and living not a mile north up Thirteenth Street.

It was classic Terri, but I tamped down a glimmering of affectionate amusement. This was serious. I took her in for a urine screen and Breathalyzer after securing her agreement to stay in her room until Faye could meet with her the next day. In what was, for Terri, unusual silence, she followed me to the bathroom, peed into the cup without protest, watched while I screwed the lid on and slid it into the plastic bag, and then sat slouched over on herself. I stripped off the gloves, tossed them into the red bag trash, and left her to a bit of privacy, reminding her to come to the nurse's office for the Breathalyzer test when she was done.

Back at the nurse's office, I prepared the Breathalyzer, a small, black box into which I inserted a disposable mouthpiece then waited for the beeping to stop and the indicator to blink the ready signal. Terri came in and sat in the chair next to the nurse's desk. I carried the instrument over to her, held it out, and reminded her—fruitlessly, as it turned out—that we'd done this before, so let's keep it simple.

As the mouthpiece came closer she began protesting again. "I ain't used, Miss Carol, I ain't used, I swear, and you ain't got to . . ."

"Terri." I used my sternest voice. She cast those big brown eyes up at me. "Just breathe into the machine. You can't do that while you're talking so much."

She did stop talking, although not in order to blow into the machine. Her breath suddenly became throttled in her throat, as though she were trying out for Camille in a very large theater with the audition committee situated in the topmost row of a high balcony.

"Give me a minute," she gurgled.

Stopped short by the really big sounds coming from the really teeny body, I stared at her. Did Terri have asthma? I didn't often remember all the women's ills and problems, but I surely would have known if she had asthma. Many of our residents did, and the nurses always told staff because there were procedures to follow if they had a crisis.

Terri, ever on the alert, took advantage of my momentary distraction by gasping, choking, and gagging between near incoherent phrases about how she couldn't breathe. Just as I snapped out of it and was about to get more heavy-handed with her, she stopped as though a voice from the wings had hissed at her about the dangers of overacting.

"No, you do not have asthma. Just breathe into the machine." I stuck it in her face, this time less patiently. Not so much because I felt impatient but because I was again tempted to laugh.

Terri thrust her neck forward and pursed her lips as though about to kiss the mouthpiece. She hitched up her shoulders, elbows akimbo, fingers outstretched. Her eyes widened, eyebrows almost disappearing into her corrugated-with-effort forehead. She placed her lips on the plastic tube. Her feet stomped a few staccato beats on the floor while she further contorted her face into an alarming expression that she must have meant as evidence of sincere, even herculean, effort. Her cheeks bulged outward, as though under great pressure. She grunted.

I almost dropped the Breathalyzer. "Terri, what the hell are you doing?"

She panted. "Trying to do the screen for you, Miss Carol. Ain't that machine felt it?"

"But you have to actually *breathe*. You have to blow breath out like you're blowing cigarette smoke. C'mon. I want to get back upstairs."

She pursed her lips, hitched her shoulders, widened her eyes, raised her eyebrows, and placed her lips on the tube. Her cheeks puffed. Her arms flailed. Her feet stomped. After a few contorted seconds she sat back in the chair and told me, "That thing must be broke if it ain't felt *that* breath."

I turned away, coughed to cover my giggles, and pretended to check the machine so as not to have to look at her. "It's not broken. You aren't breathing."

She retorted that the machine was broke and glared at it with exaggerated mistrust.

I let it go. We had the urine screen, the results of which would tell us within a day or two whether or not she'd been drinking. Just in case, I marked the form *stat* in hope the lab would send results the next morning.

"I guess I should be angry with her. But it was just so funny," I said to Tim when I got back up to the apartment, "with her eyes bugging out and her arms flapping. At least she peed. And I put a rush on the results, so we'll have them in twenty-four hours."

The results came back positive for alcohol, and Terri was yet again placed on a goals-and-behavior contract.

Meanwhile we hosted the award committee in our living room one morning in May for the final round of the competition.

A rumor floated around the house that Jackee had a boyfriend. Jessie's second grand-baby spent a Saturday with us, so thrilling the women and staff that Jessie had to tell us, more than once and with increasing crossness, to let her hold her own daughter's baby or she would smack us upside the head.

One day in June, Lawrice, Tim, Donna, Amanda, Yvonne, and I dressed up and left for the Washington Post building for the program, during which the winner of the competition would be announced. Kathy, in her final year of presidency of our board, and I had prepared the requisite presentation, she the first part and I, the second. After all five finalists had completed their presentations for the crowd of about three hundred, the committee chair announced the winner.

When they said the winning organization's name, I heard Donna shout. I noticed the people around me, Kathy included, standing and clapping. Slack jawed, I sat there staring up at Kathy, who laughed at my dumbfounded expression and hauled me to my feet.

We had won.

Wow, I thought later when, as I walked the fifteen blocks home to Miriam's House, coherent thought was finally possible. *Maybe I'm better at this job than I think I am.*

Just as I came into view a half a block away from home, a man started up from one of the patio chairs and walked swiftly away. Suspicious, I looked more closely and saw Jackee sitting there staring after the guy with an expression that could only be described as daffy.

"Awesome, he's so awesome," she said as I approached.

So began the period of Jackee's stay with us that we always refer to with two words: Awesome Al. His name, for Tim, Donna, and me at least, is forever and inextricably linked to the adjective that the love-struck Jackee used as the rest of us use an honorific. We also figured he had good reason to move swiftly away that afternoon when I first saw him. All the residents were sure he was drinking, even before he came in one evening smelling so pickled that we banned him forever from the house. Staff and residents alike counseled, cajoled, and coaxed Jackee to dump him, but her response was to keep seeing him, just farther away. She was observed on several occasions taking a full plate of food and a cup of coffee (possibly not her own food and certainly not her own plates, cups, and utensils) down the street to where he lurked, waiting for her, on the yard of an abandoned townhouse. We reprimanded her about that and about bringing his clothes in to wash in the residents' laundry room, but she was recalcitrant, so we took to inspecting every bag she brought into the house and every armful of stuff she took out of the house. If we could catch her, that is.

She herself was not drinking, at least, not according to her urine screen and Breathalyzer test results. But no one believed Awesome Al was good for her, especially given the way she had thrown over all semblance of cooperation with or interest in the community. When not plain mad at her, we worried about her. In August, Jackee announced Awesome Al had obtained an apartment, and she would move in with him. But she was so vague about the address or even in what area of the city it stood, we figured that at best he'd found space on the floor of some flop house. She moved out in August.

For a couple of weeks Jackee would come around to hang out on the patio and talk with the women, until they discovered she was gathering house gossip and telling tales to the neighbor she had befriended and on whose porch she would sit for hours at a time. The women were so upset about this they banned her from the patio altogether, none of them willing to risk her broadcasting personal information. For a few years we would see her regularly on the street for a quick chat, the focus of which was always Awesome Al. One day I realized I had not seen her for a long time. I asked around, but no one else had seen her either. None of us ever learned what had happened to Jackee.

***

"She's not like our other residents," Marge, our program director, said at staff meeting on a fall day in 2003. She was busy with a series of admission interviews with a prospective resident, Gloria, and her case manager. "She's a lot more obviously mentally ill. But I think she'll do well here, and she has a great case manager, Sara, who gives her a lot of support."

I had just told the staff that the final decision about Gloria would be the team's, but we wanted to hear their concerns as part of our deliberation.

"She's diagnosed as paranoid schizophrenic. She hears voices and sees things that aren't there. She's addicted to crack, also heroin, but seems to really want to stay sober."

Several staff member shifted uncomfortably in their chairs. I looked around the circle, watching some of the faces close. I reminded them that over the years we had become much better at living and working with mentally ill residents, that we had gained skills to help us with the Glorias of the world.

"Yeah, but *schizophrenia*?" In my peripheral vision, I could see a few heads nodding as someone spoke up. "That ain't what we have skills for."

Marge and I wanted Gloria to come in, though we knew it would be a stretch. Yvonne was unsure but willing to try. We waited to see what else would come from staff.

"It's not right to move her in and let the women deal with her. Sounds like she'd be hard to live with."

"I agree. And I'm alone on my shift at night, just me and the women. You be asleep up there. What if she freak out on my shift?"

"Or mine," added Elsie. She reminded us she had a lot to do on the evening shift—chores, dinner, cleaning up after the women, handing out the pill packets—and didn't have time to deal with someone having visions or hearing voices or whatever.

Trying to keep my voice as neutral as possible, and all the while suspecting they could see my struggle, I reminded them they were never truly alone on their shifts, even on nights and weekends. What with the in-house backup from the resident interns and me and the on-call nurse, not to mention all the notes and shift preparations, they had plenty of built-in support. But I was not convincing them, though we had been doing this for eight years. I tried again. "You personal-care aides are good at your jobs, you've gained good skills over the years, and you've handled lots of difficult situations. Give yourselves some credit."

They weren't buying it. Many PCAs tended to see a gulf between their work and mine. *You're admin, you ain't wiping their butts, you ain't on the frontline like we are.* I'd heard that time and time again. Certainly this was true, and part of me felt glad they knew they were free to say such things without repercussion. But I felt that the more germane reason was a lack of self-confidence coupled with very human reluctance to take on more work. As I saw it, these good-hearted workers had proved their abilities long ago. And I also knew that most of us fought change and worried in advance that anything or anyone new would overburden us.

Someone spoke up as though reading my mind. "You ain't got to be right there in the house, getting your hands dirty, right there with them. It's different for us."

I gave it up before I became impatient.

One of the resident interns, with the effortless competence and high self-esteem born of an upper-middle-class upbringing and education at an Ivy League school, advocated for Gloria to be admitted, reminding us we'd done it before. Plus, we could bring in someone to teach us how to work with her.

"Well," someone said, "all I know is Carol will let her in."

"It's the *team's* decision." This time I did nothing to hide my impatience. I never had grown accustomed to some staff and residents' belief that I made all the decisions all the time. "We decide together, having heard your input. And even if you don't like our decision, the things you've said make us plan better, or set up good support and training."

Silence for a few seconds. Yvonne, ready to move on, called the question. We polled the meeting, each one individually.

"I think we can manage it. Let's bring her in."

"It'll be a hell of a lot more work for some of us, but I guess we can try."

"I just want a lot of help from admin if she come."

Other staff simply nodded their assent. So we ended up bring Gloria into Miriam's House. The next year was to be hard, very hard, for all of us, yet nowhere near as hard as it was for Gloria.

CHAPTER TWENTY-SEVEN

I stood at the top of the half flight of stairs ready to welcome Gloria, who was coming up toward me dragging a large, black garbage bag stuffed with clothing. Her face was backlit by the bright springtime light pouring in the open front door, and I couldn't distinguish her features. Before I had a chance to step down to her, she had hefted that bag to her shoulder and, head down, hurried up the stairs.

I tried to introduce myself as she came level with me, but she was moving so quickly I had to jump back, grabbing the handle to the residents' hall door and jerking it open. Without a word, face still pointed downward, Gloria brushed by and followed my pointing finger into her room. She slung the heavy bag onto the floor. I stood near and waited without going in. We respected the women's need for privacy and a space safe enough to call their own. Surely Gloria, schizophrenic and paranoid, needed both more than anyone else.

"What you say your name was?" Finally, she looked up at me.

"Carol. I live here and work here, so you'll see me around a lot." I couldn't tell if she was paying attention, even though she'd asked the question. Her affect was flat, her eyes remote. I felt odd, disconnected. *Oh, dear,* I almost said aloud.

Gloria was tall, her powerful look emphasized by broad shoulders. A restless energy emanating from her in waves. She had tilted up her chin and looked down her nose when questioning me, as though peering myopically through invisible bifocals. Most remarkable, though, was that expression in her eyes and the way it made me feel.

"She's tall and big-boned, and I know she's strong because she carried that big bag up the stairs with no trouble. But I wasn't uncomfortable until she looked at me. Just about gave me the heebee-jeebees."

Tim had met her, too. "It's her eyes. They're remote. Not vacant, remote. She's in there, but not in the way you expect when you look at someone. It's internal. Haunted."

Even those of us who had advocated so strongly for Gloria to move in were a bit afraid of her. We just did not feel connected to Gloria, not when having a meal with her in the dining room, not when passing her in the hall and saying a cheerful good morning, not in any of the myriad mundane ways of living taken for granted in a small community. Gloria was disconcerting, even frightening. We eddied about her in an agitated flurry.

Even though Gloria on a good day could carry on a conversation of sorts, that expression in her eyes always held a slightly demented quality. Add the way she tilted her head and looked down her nose while speaking, and it was hard for our little community to adjust to her presence. She, more than any other of the mentally ill residents who had lived with us, projected the air of an emotionally disturbed person.

"She be creeping me out, Miss Carol. She don't belong here."

I was just happy Jessie had come to me privately, rather than bringing it up in house meeting as she usually did. "She does belong here, dear one, so I won't agree with you on that. But just like we all have things that are different or . . ."

Jessie interrupted with a look and an impatient gesture that I interpreted as *I ain't listening to one of your lectures.* But what she said was, "She be *real* different."

"Just try, Jessie. Just try." An inexpressible weariness settled over me as I watched her go and contemplated how to sort out the muddled tangle that was Gloria in our community. Or, more accurately, the muddled tangle within me now that Gloria was in our community. I almost desperately wanted her to do well, stay sober, and soften enough so that just a bit, even just a tiny bit, of our care would find entree into the fortification that was her heart.

Wasn't Gloria why we were there? For the broken ones, the misunderstood, the terribly hurt who didn't fit anywhere else? Was Gloria too unfitting even for Miriam's House? I couldn't stomach the thought and decided the community could be made to stop balking at the presence of this woman of power and vulnerability whose preyed-upon eyes watched us so closely.

"It'll work," I told myself. "Gloria is going to stay."

***

"I told you all she'd be a mess!" Elsie, just the evening before, had been the first to be confronted by Gloria having a hallucination. "Not one of you has had her come up behind you and start whispering about the dead, bloody bodies in the living room." Elsie was speaking to the group at staff meeting but looking at me. As were most of the others, while I swallowed my nerves and reminded myself this was what I'd signed up for with Gloria.

Elsie had called me the evening before, at just about eight o'clock, telling me to come down right away. She was waiting for me as I came down the stairs, barely able to hold back until we reached the privacy of my office before speaking.

"Gloria comes down the hall with her eyes bugging out. She stops and stares at me, so I ask her what's wrong. Then she tells me about the dead people she sees on the floor."

Elsie described how Gloria had stood right next to her, very close, whispering about all the bloody bodies and how she was seeing parts everywhere.

"Parts?" I asked.

"*Parts. Body* parts. *Bloody* body parts."

Assuring Elsie that she'd done the right thing in calling me, I asked where Gloria had gone. Elsie said she'd persuaded Gloria to take the medication meant for these episodes, then had taken her to her room. Elsie and I had weathered many a crisis together, so I knew she would catch her breath and go back to her usual competent, responsible work mode. I walked slowly to Gloria's room.

Gloria answered my knock in a muffled, somewhat sleepy voice. The room was dark. She was in the bed with the sheet pulled up high, the top of her head with its short-cropped, curly black hair the only part of her in view. The radio blared from its place on a shelf. I didn't ask her to turn it down because she kept it loud in order to drown out the sound of voices in her head. But the ensuing struggle to make sense of her exhausted voice and stumbling communication over the radio's noise made our conversation even more difficult.

Gloria poked her head out from underneath the sheet.

"Miss Carol. You gonna make me leave?" Shame and despair, written on her face, printed on her voice.

I assured her I wouldn't. I said she was part of the family, and I wasn't going to make her leave. We'd call Sara, whom

Gloria trusted, tomorrow. Inwardly I renewed my resolve to fight for her and hoped she could hear that in my words. She mumbled something I couldn't understand. I asked her if she could sleep, now that she'd taken the medication. She nodded without looking at me. Her glassy-eyed gaze was fixed on her sheet. Promising again we'd call Sara first thing in the morning, I told her, "We'll work it out, please don't worry." I paused.

"Don't make me go." She lifted her head off the pillow, her eyes shifting in erratic spasms about the room before dropping to her sheet once more. I wondered what she was seeing. "I ain't wanna go."

"No, no, listen to me. You'll stay. We won't make you go."

Wanting to hug her, hold her hand, or just stroke her forehead—some way to let her know I meant what I said—but refraining because Gloria didn't like to be touched, I stood in impotent silence. How could she believe me? Years of rejection and fear-induced overreactions by others in her life had presented her with too much evidence of indifference or betrayal for her to suddenly, obligingly, trust me. Powerlessness settled in my chest sharply, heavily, as though I'd breathed in iron shards.

The medications were taking effect. She was falling asleep. I tiptoed out of the room.

The next morning, afraid she'd be unwilling to get up, I knocked on her door when I came down for work. But there was no answer, so I went looking for her. I found her on the front patio, smoking the Sweet and Milds of which she was so fond. Her stare at the bricks at her feet shifted not an inch when I said good morning and asked how she was doing. I went back indoors to wait until Marge arrived.

Marge and I agreed that we needed Sara. Within a couple of hours Sara was at the house, meeting with Gloria and then with the team.

One thing we really appreciated was a good case manager, and Gloria's was one of the best I ever knew. Sara was intelligent, attentive, professional, and responsive. She shared our goal of making Gloria's residence at Miriam's House successful, and demonstrated it by being readily available to answer our questions and concerns, as well as being compassionately present to Gloria. Without her, we could not have managed to keep Gloria with us as long as we did.

This was the first of many such meetings. Sara's commitment to Gloria was beautiful. And Gloria clearly loved and trusted her. Their relationship showed us that Gloria was able to listen and respond to someone who had gained her trust. Sara also came to several staff meetings to respond to our worries and fears. She would patiently teach us about what Gloria was struggling with and show us how to support her. Dr. Bebout, her supervisor at Community Connections (a local mental-health agency) made a few hour-long training presentations about trauma-informed care. Miriam's House staff embarked on a steep learning curve. Gloria's behaviors seemed at every step to be just ahead of our knowledge, making us play catch-up for several months. It was exhausting even for me, and I could just imagine how it affected the PCAs and resident interns, who were trying to manage their already busy jobs while also dealing with Gloria.

But Gloria worked the hardest. She learned to recognize when the hallucinations were about to start, and she'd call Sara or get us to call if she couldn't. Between them, they worked out a series of small steps designed to help her understand that the voices and visions were not real. She realized that chaos in her environment made her symptoms worse, so she kept her room perfectly neat, cleaning it more often than any other resident. We bought CDs of soothing music for her to listen to as an alternative to the radio or TV. She began to participate in community life although usually waiting to be invited, appearing at Sunday breakfasts to pile a plate high, sit next to me and make monosyllabic answers to my chatter, then go outdoors for a Sweet and Mild. Though she remained mostly on the fringe and was usually silent, she did let Jessie try to interest her in the newspaper. She allowed Kimberly to hang out with her on the smokers' patio. We began to see something of the engaging, almost childish appeal Sara told us she loved so much. Awe at her courageous determination superseded the pity I had felt on the occasion of those first hallucinations.

When Gloria relapsed the first time, we were upset but not surprised. This was part of our gamble with her. Sara had explained to us that Gloria had rarely stayed sober for more than a few weeks or a month at a time. So when Marge told me one morning as I came down the stairs to my office that Gloria had not come home the night before, I was disappointed yet still somehow proud of her. She had made it three months this time, and that was a record for her as well as an indication of how committed she was to staying.

Marge and I agreed to search for her after Marge called Sara to let her know Gloria was AWOL. We got into the van and went into the areas of Northwest DC we knew were Gloria's drugging grounds, driving slowly up and down around U Street and Georgia Avenue, Sixth and O Streets, Fifth and Park Road. I sat with my face pointed out the closed window and craning my neck for a glimpse of her.

"If she used last night," Marge said, sounding defeated after we'd been driving a while and not seen Gloria, "she's probably in some crack house, sleeping it off. Probably not out on the street at all right now." But she didn't stop driving and I didn't stop looking.

Needle in a haystack, I thought, then asked if we knew what she was wearing.

"No, but probably that rag."

We smiled. Gloria, whose close-trimmed hair allowed her to wear skullcaps and bandanas, had a favorite piece of fabric she'd tie around her head, a not-so-distinctive black, but it gave us something to look for: a tall, rangy woman with a particular look in her eye and a black do-rag tied about her head.

It didn't help. We never saw her. We drove back to Miriam's House to find out whether she'd called Sara or the house, but she had not. I went to my office and fell into my chair. How could riding around in a van for an hour be so exhausting?

I made sure her front-door key card was deprogrammed. I typed the sign for the front door, the sign I posted whenever a resident went AWOL:

If Gloria comes to the door, do not let her in.

Get staff.

In the meanwhile, let's pray for her.

Two days later, Gloria contacted Sara. When Marge came and told me that Sara was on her phone, I went to her office so that, with Sara on speaker, we could work out our next steps.

"She admits to smoking crack. She's pretty broken up about it, Carol. She really wants to try again at Miriam's House."

We had never discharged a resident for a first relapse, or even a second or sometimes not even a third, and weren't about to start with Gloria, I assured Sara, as long as she brought no drugs or alcohol into the house. We mostly felt relieved to know where she was. It was time to work out the logistics of getting her back and finding ways to better support her.

We agreed that Gloria needed something stricter than our boilerplate goals-and-behavior contract. We modified it so that each of the four stages lasted four weeks instead of the usual two. We delayed the date at which she'd gain permission to go out by herself, and even then gave her a four o'clock cur-few instead of six o'clock. As I left the office and Marge began planning for Gloria's return, I realized I felt nowhere near the confidence I'd communicated, just the same determination to make it so she could stay.

But as that summer wore on, Gloria relapsed again and then again, each time managing a shorter interval of sobriety before succumbing once more to the addiction. A group that included Sara, Marge, Yvonne, and me, and often her mother, met regularly to check in with Gloria, monitor her progress and her moods, and devise and redevise a program that would work for her. We instituted unprecedented measures, all of them worked out with Gloria's input and agreement: earlier curfews than usual, less freedom of movement, additional sup-port groups and counseling. Yet she continued to relapse. We were running out of ideas. The other residents were becom-ing nervous about living with someone who could not remain sober. There grew a palpable tension in our little community.

Gloria herself ended it all. She broke the one no-compromise rule by bringing crack into the house and smok-ing it in her room. It wasn't that she didn't understand. Gloria was smart and could figure out the bottom line. But the addic-tion was so strong and the state of her mental health so debili-tating that sobriety was not only too hard for her, it simply held no attraction. Sober, Gloria was assured of frightening visual and aural hallucinations that she'd learned early in life to ban-ish with street drugs. Whatever else smoking crack did, at least it eased those violent, bloody visions, smothered the urgently insistent, disembodied voices, and made her feel she had some power over them.

I came to wonder if her decision to break a cardinal rule was her way of telling us she was not capable of living at Miriam's House.

***

Miriam's House was not for everyone. I said this often, as a way to remind all of us that the work we were doing, good and needed work though it may have been, was not the end-all and be-all for every woman with AIDS in DC. In retrospect, I realized that I'd never said it about Gloria. I'd never stepped back from my single-minded determination to keep her with us in order to ask whether Miriam's House was truly the best place for her. As a result, after she herself made it so startlingly clear, I was left wondering if I had not been a party to what pushed her to it.

We had long before created an application process that allowed time and space for both Miriam's House and the prospective resident to discover if the fit was good. And the question about fit also applied when women already living with us were struggling. Our practice was to have an open, inclusive exploration of what was best for the resident. Her case manager and family would participate in meetings with Miriam's House staff and the struggling woman herself. Most often this process resulted in the resident's renewed determination and us having formed a more solid support system for her. And the process itself was open enough to leave little room for any one person's manipulation. Perhaps knowing about the open-ended quality of these investigations made me subconsciously reject beginning it in Gloria's case. Understandable. And yet.

And yet, I had to wonder if I had not been unfair to Gloria. Would things have turned out differently had I been willing to call a special meeting so we could engage the question about fit? I couldn't know. But I could wonder because I knew that unless we caregivers were willing to be scrupulously honest about our inner motives and needs, we could do a disservice to the very persons we were charged to protect.

***

The phone rang one evening when I was nursing a migraine, and even as I picked it up, I knew.

"Carol, the residents tell me they smell crack outside Gloria's room. They're really upset."

I sped downstairs, headache ignored for the time being, although I knew I'd pay for it later. Jessie, Kimberly, and several others were waiting for me at the bottom of the stairs on the first floor. I slowed down and stepped into the swirl of panicked, angry voices.

"Miss Carol, it ain't right!"

"She making me feel sick. I can't be smelling that shit."

"I share that bathroom with her, can smell crack clear as if I be in the crack house. Ain't staying here if you gonna let bitches be smoking up in here."

"Get her out."

I stood and listened, nodding occasionally and looking at each one in turn until they wound down. "I know, I know. I'll go to Gloria. How about you get to the dining room or TV room? Away from the smell. Call your sponsors if you need to, we don't need a double relapse. Where's Elsie? She can hang out with you for a while."

Watching them go past me, touching each on the hand or shoulder, I steeled myself for what was ahead.

I knocked on Gloria's door. She mumbled something and I went in. She was crouched over in the chair in what would have been a fetal position were she lying down.

"You've been smoking crack, Gloria."

A nod. Her head and neck drooped toward the floor. She did not lift her face to me, she did not look up. Not once while I was in that room did our eyes meet.

"Give me the pipe." I took it from her. "Give me the bag." I took it from her.

"Where did you smoke it?" She made a quick gesture toward the half bath shared with her next-door neighbor. I went in, looked around, saw nothing, and went back to her to ask if she had any more in the room or in her purse. A shake of the head. Still I picked up the purse and shook it out. Nothing, Looked on top of the dresser, bedside table, the bed, the closet. Nothing. Stood in the middle of that immaculately tidy room and saw—nothing. But I didn't walk away. I stood. Finally I said, softly, that I had to call Sara. She nodded. I told her she must agree to stay in her room, the PCAs would check regularly about food and drink. "In the morning we'll meet with you, just try to get some sleep now." She nodded, one slight bob of her head at each instruction, eyes fixed to the floor, still huddled in the chair.

I left. Finally, I left her.

Sara found Gloria a place in one of the Community Connection semi-independent group homes. Gloria moved out, leaving a hole in our home and in me.

She visited several times that fall after I called her and invited her to Sunday breakfast, which she had always loved. She'd show up late, serve herself a heaping plate of food, and sit at the table with me, forcing out a quick word or two in answer to my comments and questions. Then, restless as ever, she would be on her way. We continued to hope for her. But one day Sara told us Gloria had left her program. A few days later, as Tim and I drove down Florida Avenue and crossed Georgia, we saw her hanging out on a corner we knew was her habitual drugging area. By the time we'd realized it was her, and Tim had found a safe place to turn the car around, she had disappeared. We never saw Gloria again.

We lost touch with Sara until, a year or so later, she called us with the news that Gloria had overdosed and died.

The temptation was to decry the hours in training, the meetings with Sara and Dr. Bebout, the effort we put into making Gloria's stay with us a success, and conclude that all had been for naught. On the surface, that was true. Nothing we had done seemed to have made much of a difference.

Except that Gloria had the experience, during what turned out to be her final year of life, of living in a loving, accepting, safe community and of gaining a bit of self-esteem by overcoming some of her demons.

Except that Miriam's House was a stronger organization, better equipped, and more confident to welcome women with serious mental-health issues.

Except that Miriam's House staff was somehow more open, having learned to love one who initially had seemed far more frightening than lovable. Those hours spent in meetings and trainings may not have had the ultimate effect we longed for—Gloria's sobriety and long life at Miriam's House—yet they'd had the effect of beginning a transformation in us. This came about only after long discussions and fielding numerous resident complaints. And who could blame us? In Gloria's case, our fears of her were just as understandable and just as real as her mistrust and fear of us. That made it all the more wonderful that she eventually grew to feel more at home with us, as did we with her.

Gloria's legacy was this: she made Miriam's House a better place. She did this by trying harder than she ever had in all her life to live clean and fight the schizophrenia. Her gutsy choice to resist the ultimate temptation of crack, thus assuring a return of the plague of visions and voices, was amazing beyond words. Her legacy was to make it so that other women like her, whom we would have been unable to welcome before, could come into Miriam's House and find what was often the first loving, fully accepting home they'd ever had.

This woman who was homeless, paranoid schizophrenic, subject to traumatic visions and frantic voices, helplessly addicted to crack, living with AIDS, and dead at the age of thirty-five, showed us what courage is.

CHAPTER TWENTY-EIGHT

"Carol, Washington Hospital Center just called about Jessie. She's acting up again."

Yvonne and I exchanged knowing and perhaps weary glances.

"What happened this time?"

"She pressed the button for the nurse but I guess decided she'd waited too long, so she hauled her stubborn self out of the bed, down the hallway, and threw herself on the floor in front of the nurses' station."

I tried not to smile, but failed. "That is *so* Jessie."

"Yeah, well, they want someone to come talk with her."

That would be me. For one thing, Yvonne was the only nurse on staff at that time, and was needed at the house. And for some reason Jessie listened to me. This had to do with my being the executive director, Jessie being respectful, or fearful, of people with power. But it also had to do with our boundless patience with and affection for each other.

I left for the hospital.

***

Coming up to her room, I knocked on the door and poked my head in.

"Hey, Miss Carol!"

We hugged, awkwardly, Jessie reaching her arms up and me bending over the bed. Sitting down on the space she cleared for me amidst the tangle of sheets, food wrappers, straws, and juice boxes, I told her some of the Miriam's House news. She asked about each resident one by one. After a bit, I got to the point of this visit.

"You know, the hospital called us."

She scrunched her body higher in the bed and adjusted the pillows behind her back, round face puckered in a frown that dragged her face to the center like a pouch with the drawstring pulled tight. "Miss Carol, I ain't done nothing! They don't never come when I buzz. Act like they don't care, always talking about having other patients.

The IV lines, several of them snaking down from multiple bags hanging on the pole next to and looming above her bed, had tangled in the repositioning. She plucked at them impatiently, angrily, muttering under her breath, "Damn things, can't hardly move."

She looked up. "I done pressed that buzzer a half a hour ago and ain't nobody come yet. That nurse don't care about me."

She had been seven years on kidney dialysis, seven years of four-hour, three-times-per-week periods of immobility at a medical facility that smelled of ammonia and something else unnameable and sickly powerful. She had survived with scars, some of which were visible on her face and body, left by a husband with a predilection for mean ways with sharp knives. And she had, I knew from my own efforts to explain things to her, limited cognitive abilities.

"And I ain't had fresh ice water or nothing yet today."

I said I'd get her water and ice. "Jessie, how have you been treating the nurses?"

"I been treating 'em fine, Miss Carol." But her tone was peevish, with none of the righteous indignation of the wrongly accused.

"Really?"

"Well, but she be rough. And take so long to get here."

"Come on, Jessie, how do you expect people to treat you when you treat them badly?"

"They ain't never *that* nice to me."

"You know what I mean."

The television was making annoying, loudly insistent claims on our attention. Jessie was quiet for a moment, face turned toward the window and a bright blue and lovely winter sky. We waited. Head still turned away so that I was looking at her profile, she talked about how sick her mother was and blind and that made Jessie wish she could help out more, how being in the hospital so much made her sad, how the girls— *You know I love 'em but four teenagers be a shitload a trouble—* haven't called her since she ain't know when.

I know when but forbore to remind her. They mainly called Jessie near the first of the month when her disability check was in and they knew she had money. And they called when they were in trouble.

"And now they having babies. I tell you yet the second one pregnant? And I love me my grandbabies but, God . . ." She shook her head. "I can't take it sometimes."

We were again silent in the stream of noise out of the television hanging from the ceiling by a long, elbowed, metal arm. In a moment, she picked up the theme again, upset that ain't none of them doctors American, and who could understand them accents? And how creepy when they gathered around the bed, standing over and talking past her sometimes without really looking at her and then acted like she ain't have the right to ask questions.

"And I ain't understand them big words, Miss Carol, I ain't understand none of it."

I could barely hear her next words, they were spoken so low, and Jessie was still turned, unseeing, toward the window.

"I ain't know what's wrong with me."

Wishing violently that a doctor were with us to hear this, I, too, looked toward the window for a time before I spoke. She said yes when I asked her if she wanted to know what was wrong, so I called Yvonne back at the house. Yvonne assured Jessie she'd connect with Jessie's primary doctor as soon as she could, then interpret the diagnoses and concerns to her.

"Thanks, Miss Yvonne." Jessie replaced the receiver. Her face sagged. She plucked at the IV lines.

"Jessie," I reached out for her hand, the one without the IV lines coming out of the nasty looking bruise on her arm, "we want you to get good care here, get better, and come home. The trip to Six Flags is coming up soon."

"Can't go anyway with dialysis."

I assured Jessie that Amanda had scheduled the trip on a Saturday so she could go. She smiled and promised to be better. She wanted to get to Six Flags.

***

"I don't hold out much hope that Jessie will ever really change, but she can behave better with regular reminders," I told Yvonne upon my return from the hospital, "and it makes me uncomfortable to speak to her so maternally. I just haven't found anything else that works."

So much had changed in me since those early years of anxiety, strained relationships, hurt feelings, and noncomprehension. Here was where I first felt the difference most clearly, in my ability to deal with Jessie. Along the way the women had taught me to be genuine instead of needy. They'd taught me to love them without agenda. In the space freed up by authenticity and love, I'd learned to meet each woman where she was. I could set aside (for the most part—I was never perfect at any of this) my ego and needs in order to just be there. The sternness that I often had to employ had been gained during these years of arduous professional experience and was firmly rooted in compassion. The difference this balance afforded me was astounding, as I compared current interactions with Jessie to long-ago interactions with Tamara and Janelle. There would always be more to learn, and most of it about myself, but compassion, inner peace, and increasing gratitude were the fruits of my labors. What more could I want?

Yet I knew I was seen as spoiling Jessie. Later on, while other staff came regularly to the point of demanding she be discharged, I probably seemed just as stubborn as she did. But short of sending her to a nursing home, for which we were not sure she qualified anyway, there was nowhere else for Jessie to go. Not that I was looking.

Anyway, that hospital visit ended well. Meaning no more theatrical collapses at the nurses' station.

**

Kimberly had relapsed a couple of times again soon after the drunken Christmas 1996 incident, but otherwise had done well with us, her quirky ways both accepted and treated warily by residents and staff. But by midsummer 2004, her behavior became harder for staff to manage. We tried to work things out in our usual ways. We held compassion meetings with her and support meetings with staff, counselor, and sister. We levied consequences, drove her to counseling appointments, asked her to take on responsibilities that, we hoped, would bring out the maturity we knew was in her somewhere.

Instead of responding positively as she had in the past, she began fighting with staff in a way that we'd not heard or seen from her in nine years. Her urine screens were clean, so we were pretty sure she wasn't drinking, although she certainly was acting as though she were. She refused to attend doctor appointments. She skipped her counseling and psychiatric visits. Her erratic behavior continually wreaked havoc in our sensitive community, and even with all our resources at her service, it got worse. She loudly and profanely accused one of the PCAs of stealing her purse, upsetting him so much he called me in to search for it and was triumphantly vindicated when I found it under her bed. She and Jessie, who had fought off and on since Jessie moved in but always made up to go back to being best friends, came to blows with fist and key chain one evening after house meeting. Everything we knew to do—get her a mental-health counselor, monitor how she took her medications, meet with her, meet with her and her sister, meet with her and her sister and her counselor—she fought as though we were asking her to do herself physical harm. Finally, with both reluctance and relief, we decided Kimberly needed a change after nine years with us. We arranged for transfer to another facility, aided by the DC Long-Term Care Ombudsman Program's Lydia Williams, who began advocating for Kimberly as soon as we'd said we might need to transfer her.

Lydia was a practical, strong woman who commanded instant respect. She did not sugar-coat but, with as few and as strong words as possible, outlined a resident's alternatives to her and our responsibilities to us. She was a wonderful advocate for the women. Most of them responded well to her and allowed her to work with them and the staff in order to resolve the issues and stay at Miriam's House. For some reason, Kimberly would not or could not respond in this way. But she also would not agree to move to another facility, telling us all to go to hell. She chose to move in with her stepmother, which meant returning to the house and the neighborhood in which she had first begun drinking as a teenager.

Appalled, we argued strenuously against this move. But Kimberly had made the choice, as was her right. One night in early December 2004, she left without ceremony, without telling us, and without taking much with her. She called me later in the week, not, as I hoped when I heard the familiar rough voice, to ask to come home, but to find out if she could come get the rest of her things. She and I made arrangements for her to attend our Christmas party the next night, after which we would load up the van and I would drive her across town to her Northeast neighborhood.

Once again, Christmas time. Once again, Kimberly and I together and at odds.

❆❆❆

I drove slowly. The roads had frozen spots, and the snow that was still falling made blurred patches of the pavement ahead. I asked Kimberly how she was doing in her new home.

"I be fine, Miss Carol, you ain't got to worry."

But I heard a lack of conviction in her voice. I probed a bit. "Do you spend much time with your stepmom?"

"Nah. She work."

"Is the house nice?"

"Yeah, she keep it nice." The gruff voice was low, uncertain.

"Where do you sleep?"

"Couch."

"I thought there was a basement with a room and a bed. What happened to that?" I hated the idea of a couch-surfing Kimberly.

She looked down and paused. "A man stay down there, but I ain't like him."

"Why not?"

"He drink."

"Oh, Kimberly." I concentrated on my driving, noting how unshed tears make shimmering stars of traffic and Christmas lights.

"I be fine, Miss Carol. Don't worry about me. I ain't want to drink again. Don't worry."

We pulled into a parking space off the alley behind the house and got out, each of us grabbing a bag or two. Kimberly produced the house key. No one was home and we quickly carried in the rest of the bags so as to get out of the drifting cold. I looked around at the tiny house, each room and each flat surface holding signs of life lived long in place: photos stained orange with age of people in Sixties-era clothing, souvenirs of Ocean City, and plastic angels in attitudes of prayer. Scattered among these objects were Santas and elves and more angels, these with devout expressions and outstretched arms.

"See? I'll be fine."

I wasn't sure whom she was trying to persuade.

***

Amid the disruption around Kimberly's leaving, we continued preparations for holidays the thought of which made me feel a lot more fatigued than festive. The women, unnerved by the sight of Kimberly out of control and then gone, flocked to the Bible study taught by a volunteer pastor most Monday nights.

In the midst of my small funk, my brother, Bill, called with an idea for Christmas. He wanted to send presents to the residents. We worked out a plan whereby Bill would buy sweaters for each woman in the color and size of her choice. Amanda wrote up a list of the women's choices that I then e-mailed to Bill. He called me a week or so later to say he'd been shopping.

"I showed the saleswomen the list of what I wanted, and they got all excited. Helped me for an hour, double-checked the list to make sure we had the right color with the right size. They say Merry Christmas to everyone."

When the three large boxes packed with gift bags arrived the week before Christmas, Donna and I cut carefully through the packing tape and pulled out a couple of the bags with their matching tissue paper and ribbons tied to the handles.

"Now I'm getting into the Christmas spirit," said Donna, trying in vain to peek through the paper.

***

Elsie motioned to me from the doorway of the nurse's office. She and I had done Christmas Eve together for all of the seven years she's worked at Miriam's House. We had our own little traditions and habits, including acting like big kids ourselves.

"Is everything ready for us elves to get started?"

We grinned at each other like the coconspirators we were. "A lot of the women are still up." I looked at the clock. "It's past eleven. We shouldn't wait too much longer."

"Let's at least put the stockings by the doors. And if they're still up after that, we'll just take the presents in under the tree. It'll still be a surprise."

While Elsie distracted the women in the living room and dining room, I began the Stocking Placement.

Stealth was my watchword. I wouldn't surprise the women if they saw or heard me in the hallway lugging a box full of stockings. My strategy was designed to get them placed without anyone noticing. I pictured the women coming out of their rooms or opening the hall door and seeing the stockings on parade near each door down the hall.

I opened the door to the residents' first-floor wing, wondering why the wrapping paper only seemed to rustle so loudly when I needed it to be quiet. I tiptoed. At each door, it was the same routine. Pause to listen if anyone was coming, put box on floor, lift out stocking, place in optimal position beside door— in view, but not in the way—and sneak to the next door.

First floor, seven doors. No one saw me. I took the back stairway down to the ground floor and repeated, then the same stairs up to the second floor. Repeat.

It didn't take long. It was silly, maybe even a tad childish, but I enjoyed thinking I'd managed it in secret. Surely the women in their rooms heard me and were, even as I glided off their floor and onto the next, opening their doors and pulling those stockings in for a thorough dismantling.

Back in the dining room, I nodded significantly to Elsie. The women were still hanging around, one or two in the kitchen and the rest in the living room with the lights off and the tree on, music playing. We strolled with studied nonchalance to my office where the presents awaited distribution.

Many pairs of eyes watched attentively as we went back and forth with presents, putting them under and around the tree. It took several trips. We brought in Bill's bags last.

"Do we wait till tomorrow to open these?"

"It's up to you," Elsie said.

We all sat there while Terri cast longing glances at the gift bags. Finally she said, "I just want to know which is mine."

She got up from the couch and bent over a bag. "Nope, not mine." She took a step toward another bag.

"Hey! Ain't right to just look for yours!"

"Yeah, go back, girl, and see who gets that one."

"What are you gonna do? Open it now? Don't you want to be surprised in the morning?"

"Just about morning now. Whose bag is that one? I couldn't hear her."

"Tamika."

"Tamika, your bag that one in the front! You gonna look in it?"

"Are we allowed to?" She looked at me.

I ignored the feeling of dismay that rose with that look. "Really, it's up to you, each of you. I can't tell you how to celebrate Christmas."

"Well, I ain't opening no presents now. We should wait for Christmas Day, like after breakfast or something.

"Fine, you wait. I'm getting mine now. Seems close enough to Christmas already."

"Yeah, it do."

Terri and most of the others waded into the sea of presents under the tree, bumping into one another and calling out names, handing bags over shoulders until all that wanted to were sitting down with Bill's bags in their laps.

Now what?

"I ain't want to open it now, I just wanted to look at it."

"What good does that do?"

"Gets me excited for Christmas."

Terri's forefinger was quietly, busily poking a hole in the tissue paper peeking out of the top of her bag.

"I'm already plenty excited."

"The music stopped, someone go put another CD on."

"Why don't you? We ain't taking orders from you."

"I can't make that machine work."

Terri's finger had worked its way through the layers of tissue paper. She pulled it out of the hole she'd made and peered in.

"I'll put one in. And get a snack. What we got left over from dinner?"

"Some of that macaroni and cheese is left, I think. I want some too, bring me a plate. Not here," suddenly remembering the rule about eating in the living room and throwing a hurried look at Elsie's face, "in the dining room. We'll eat in the dining room."

The hole was too tiny and the light from the tree too dim for Terri to see the contents of her bag. She slowly and carefully peeled back more of the tissue paper, revealing soft yellow material.

"Dang, Terri done opened hers! Ain't it pretty?"

The sight of that splash of color seemed to unleash a torrent as every woman with a bag on her lap dove in and began tearing. The floor was soon awash in paper and discarded gift bags, the air with a swell of voices going on about color and size and *perfect!* Women held up sweaters and even matching turtlenecks we had not expected. I blinked hard, quite still amidst the profusion of paper and tinsel and twinkle lights and joy.

* * *

For a few weeks during the holidays Kimberly talked with Donna and me by phone and chatted with the women at the day program, giving them messages to bring home to us. Then, just after the first of the year, she dropped out of sight. Rumor had it she was drinking, but no one actually saw her.

In early February 2005 we finally had information about her when a social worker at Washington Hospital Center called. She said Kimberly was on life support in the intensive-care unit.

Perhaps Kimberly made poor choices in those last months of her life. We didn't know why, but we knew that many residents began behaving erratically as they aged. The long-term effects of AIDS, its toxic medications, and their own history of drug and alcohol abuse took a toll on their brains. It seemed that Kimberly's choices to leave us and, we believed, to begin drinking again had led directly to her death. We couldn't know with any certainty.

But what was certain was that I was standing again at the bedside of a dying woman, and she beloved of me. What was certain was that this woman and all the others who deserved the best of this world had, instead, received the scraps. I had once imagined we could live forever, that our life together at Miriam's House would never end. But it did end, and far too often it did so at the bedside of a woman too young, who had so much to teach us but instead was dying in near anonymity. And so I wished, not for the first time, to find a way for them to be heard and known so that others might love and value them as they deserved.

Kimberly had said to me many times over the nine years she'd been with us, "You know, I'd be dead now if it wasn't for Miriam's House." That phrase went through my head as I stood there listening to the steady hissing and pumping of the ventilator. I had always responded the same way, as I did to every woman who expressed a similar sentiment to me: "All we can do is hold out for you the opportunity to choose a different life. Your own strength and courage make it work for you."

We could not know why or how Kimberly had ended up in the ICU dependent upon a machine for her life. But what we could know was that Kimberly had the fortitude and willpower to live well those nine years with us. She'd battled the disease as well as guilt for passing it on to her son, and worked dauntlessly to overcome her addiction while living in a community of women all consumed with similar struggles. That she managed so long and so well overshadows the lapses of her final months. All Miriam's House did was hold out the opportunity to her. Kimberly's own strength and courage had made it work.

Always, and for each of these women, it was what was within them that made Miriam's House work.

EPILOGUE

Kimberly's funeral was crowded with her family and child-hood friends, her twelve-step buddies, people from the women's groups she attended, and all of us from Miriam's House. We arrived a bit late and so had to sit in a side balcony from where we could see Kimberly's sister and other family member in the front pew. And there was Jamal. That was what got to us. Seeing Jamal.

But our tears dried in horror when one of the women's HIV/AIDS group leaders stood up to talk about Kimberly. Maybe she honestly didn't know that Kimberly had never told her family she was living with AIDS. Maybe she wanted to break the silence and diffuse the cloud of shame that still, in 2005, enshrouded the disease. For whatever reason, she announced that she had first met Kimberly in her group for women with AIDS. We could barely breathe. I wanted to jump up and shout at her to shut up, it's not her right to out Kimberly. I didn't dare look at Jamal.

With Kimberly gone, Terri seemed to become even less committed to the tenuous hold she had on sobriety and health. After getting an apartment with her boyfriend, John, she dropped from sight for months at a time, calling Donna after longer and longer intervals to hear the gossip and find out how everyone was. She never asked to come home. I saw her one last time, in 2007, when she called me from Providence Hospital emergency room where she'd brought John, who was in crisis. I drove over to be with her. She paced nervously, worried about John, so unwilling to look me in the eye that I figured she was high. At some point later that year, she entered Joseph's House, by then strictly a hospice for people with cancer and AIDS. Being Terri, she defied the doctor's expectations and got better instead of dying. After she left Joseph's House, we didn't hear from her at all, not even a call to Donna. She died a few months later, alone and on the street, living the life she would not abjure, the life that killed her.

That was the thing about Miriam's House. You had to keep giving it permission to break your heart.

Jessie stayed with us until her death in October 2008. Whenever her struggle to contain her frustration and anger failed her, I'd tell her I'd have to call adult emergency services to have her taken out of Miriam's House. She'd promise to be good. She'd say she didn't want to leave and she would stop. Which she always did, until the next time. And I didn't care, if it kept her with us.

In the end, she died during what had seemed to be the typical hospital stay with the typical complaints she had always before overcome. Knowing my migraines were bad, she told me just to call her instead of visiting. *I be fine, Miss Carol, you just take care of yourself.* With some gratitude, I took her advice. And so, when she died alone in the hospital one night, I had not visited her at all, had not understand how ill she was, and was not with her as she breathed her last.

And that was another thing about Miriam's House. It always needed more from me than I could ever give it. Over the years I had come to terms with the feeling that the needs were too much, the resources—mine and the world's—too few, energy and will in too short supply. Was it ego that had made me think I could do it all? I thought it probably was. Pride, the need to be perfect, the best. Well, I was not the best and had proved that to myself many times. Jessie represented one more woman I had let down. I had to make my peace with that.

Jessie had planned to do the Fannie Mae Help the Homeless Walkathon with us that November. In her memory, I walked the five miles pushing her wheelchair with her favorite doll strapped into the seat, its head bobbing with the bumpy ride. We crossed the finish line, Dora the Explorer and me, next to Marcie, who had walked the whole way despite having lost a lung to surgery in July. I was so proud of Marcie and she of herself that we hugged, laughing and pounding each other on the back. Then I straightened up Dora, who had flopped over in the excitement, my joy fading as I fished a tissue out of my pocket.

Faye, Donna, Elsie, Yvonne, Tim, and I worked together until I had to leave. Over the years, the migraines had gradually become more and more debilitating, and I finally admitted to myself I was unable to continue the work I loved. In August 2009, I presented my resignation to the board of directors, effective December 31. Using the succession plan I had written some years before, we all prepared for my leaving. I knew it was the right thing to do. The women deserved better than I had been able to give them for the past year or two. Still, knowing it was right provided only small comfort.

***

December 31, 2009: my final shift at Miriam's House. The
women and I saw the new year in together, munched on
brownies and chips, and cheered for 2010. They'd said good
night. Some said good-bye, although Tim and I were not to
move out until February.

I made my nighttime circuit around Miriam's House, the
same route I'd walked throughout fourteen years of duty nights
and walk-throughs. Leaving my office, where I'd written my logbook notes, I turned left and entered the first-floor residents'
wing. There in the room to my left was Tamara, sprawled on
the floor and applying lipstick, and to my right, Gloria, lying in
bed with the covers over her face and listening to quiet music.
Next to her, Little Karen groaned and choked while her mother
wept. Farther down the hall, and I stood between the room
where Nickie fought for breath while Kathy prepared to do
CPR, and the room where Miss Doris watched her new television. Across from the back staircase was Terri, complaining,
trying to show Linda and me her . . . condition.

As always, I went down the back stairway, remembering
the crunch of empty syringes under my shoes when I first
walked through the building in 1993. On the ground-floor
residents' wing, I passed the mechanical room where I first
learned how the building systems worked, then the rec room at
the end of the hall, listening to echoes of meetings and smelling pizza. I opened the staff lounge door, turning off the light
in the room where Faye and I first squared off before risking
friendship, where we met with residents in compassion meetings, and from which we staged parties because even with the
huge kitchen upstairs we still needed the extra space, the stove,
and the oven. The laundry room, painted yellow in recent years
and so much more cheerful, was tidy. The light was off in the
storage room where I once searched for a radio for Janelle's
bath, where we stored the artificial Christmas tree and all the

ornaments and decorations, and where Tim kept the tools and supplies for his maintenance work.

I retraced my steps to the front stairs and there was Sasha, her head down and her step heavy. Rebecca was being wheeled out the front door, her head also down. Jessie and Kimberly were on the smokers' patio, arguing loudly about something that would not, could not, ruin their friendship. Then Tamara was walking toward me—*I'm home!*

I turned from the front door and saw coming down the stairs two grave, black-suited men in white gloves, gently maneuvering a stretcher on which lay a long, zippered bag. I made way for Gloria, who wanted no help after heaving to her shoulder the black twenty-gallon bag stuffed with her life.

To the left, into the hallway to look at the photos lining the wall before opening the kitchen door to the clattering of pots and popping of frying foods and warnings about *What I'ma do to the bitch who stole my bacon,* and *Hey, Muriel, these beans is done, you want some?* I smelled Kimberly's fried bologna and Tamara's chitlins and Jessie's crabs.

And there in the dining room was Gina/Sha-nay-nay, wobbling about and exuding Attitude. Crystal, unable to see her, laughed anyway and then wondered aloud who would read her to sleep. Terri came through the door in a T-shirt and hiking boots and poked fun at Muriel, who was slapping her knife down on some hard-ass waffles. Gloria sat in the corner, watching, eyes wary.

From beneath the noise rose the sound of voices from fourteen years of meals and parties and bingo games and funeral repasts.

Passing through to the living room, I saw the chairs circled for house meeting, the women slung onto them and the sofas with varying degrees of patience and attention. Tim held up an empty beer can, Donna reminded the women that the sanitizer was not a dishwasher. I said, as I had so often, that there was nowhere else I wanted to be. Rebecca started to cry. I looked again and the chairs were circled for a memorial service, and the low table in the center was covered with a purple-print shawl on which sat a photo, a candle, tea lights, and a Bible. Behind me, a Christmas tree's tinsel glistened in the colored lights.

In the TV room, Kimberly had the television volume too loud, and I told her to turn it down. Before retracing my steps down the kitchen hallway, I looked back once more and saw several of the women with Elsie and Terri, watching a gospel music show, or maybe it was the BET awards.

Down the kitchen hallway I heard Faye cooking Sunday dinner, singing with the gospel music playing on the din- ing-room stereo. Kathy came out of the nurses' office and reminded me that I don't get to choose. Donna passed me with latex gloves on her hands, prepared for monthly room inspec- tions. Elsie beckoned me from the nurse's office, *Ready to be the Christmas elves?* Yvonne calmly instructed someone how to use the blood-sugar tester. I heard the tap-tap of shoes on the floor as Terri choked into a Breathalyzer.

Back again to the front stairway and up to the second floor. Alyssa's room door opened and Brianna tiptoed out, *She sleep.* I stopped outside Kimberly's room to sniff for cigarette smoke, and outside Latrice's, where Faye organized our Christmas presents for return to Ames.

That's all. After returning to my office for the final sign-off on the daily logbook, I went to my apartment. Turning around for a final survey of the hallway, I saw, leaning against the wall outside of every door, fourteen years' worth of stockings, Mother's Day gifts, Easter baskets, and Valentine presents I'd placed there. I heard Alyssa's gospel music, Jessie's television, the sounds of a PCA's bucket and mop, the shower running, and Kimberly's gruff voice, *Well, well*. I saw us, very early and in the dark one morning, disappearing into the room where a woman lay with hands crossed on her still chest.

I closed my apartment door.

***

It's late winter 2010, and Tim and I are settled into a rented house in Mount Pleasant, close enough for Tim that his walk to work is only fifteen minutes. Far enough away for me that there are no constant reminders, except those in my own mind. We've bought a used glider chair on Craigslist and put it in the second-floor sunroom that overlooks roof and treetop to the woods near the zoo. It starts to snow almost as soon as we move in, the storm named Snowmageddon smoothing white the world while I rock and grieve. Finally, impelled by an impulse barely acknowledged, I get up. I go to the office where Tim set up the computer I've been avoiding for weeks. I begin to type:

This is what I remember most vividly about Kimberly . . .

AUTHOR'S NOTE

I relied on daily log notes, my journal, my memory, and the memories of former staff members and residents for the stories in this memoir. All conversations are reconstructed, although several of my early readers and I can vouch for the authenticity of their subject matter and voice, especially those of staff meetings and resident gatherings. Some names have been changed, especially of those Miriam's House residents now dead, who were very private about their health status when they were alive.

ACKNOWLEDGMENTS

Without the women of Miriam's House, this memoir would not be. My primary acknowledgments are to them and to how their power of example influenced and changed me. This book is theirs.

If you have read the book, you know Tim, my wonderful husband. I do not exaggerate his good qualities; indeed, I hold back my praise of him. But by now you know that without the support and love of this good, kind, intelligent, and caring man, my work at Miriam's House would not have been possible. My deepest love and best gratitude are for Tim Fretz.

The foundations for my work came in my early years, when my parents taught me the values on which I founded Miriam's House: hard work, integrity, commitment, and responsibility. My father died in 2006, and his name is in the dedication of this book. My mother is alive and, at eighty-six years old, indomitable. She trains a German shepherd dog, showing it in obedience trials and often winning. They raised entrepreneurs, three of their four children having founded and run their own businesses. I am grateful for their example.

Special thanks go to my sister, Joan Marsh Sparks, who read early chapters with encouragement and understanding, and whose business acumen greatly benefitted my Inkshares preorder campaign. To Joan and to her colleague and my friend, Kristen Michelle, who also gave unstinting advice, I want to express warmest love and gratitude.

Sometimes you find a friend who is more than a friend, who is simpatico in a way that enriches and challenges you. Such a friend is Juliana Bateman. Her encouragement is unflagging, and her thoughts and advice on sections of this book were invaluable.

Special thanks are due to the Goucher College community of writers in the Master of Fine Arts in Creative Nonfiction program. Patsy Sims built a strong and communal program. And my mentors, each in their own way, deeply influenced this book, which was my master's thesis. Suzannah Lessard tamed my overly sentimental and wandering writing style, striking whole paragraphs with a decisive slash of her pencil. Richard Todd guided the trajectory of the book, focusing me deeper in story and reflection. Diana Hume George directed the manuscript with empathy for the women and brilliant, unsentimental advice for me. During my fourth semester, I studied the essay form with Jacob Levinson, whose intellectual and intuitive approach to writing informs me to this day.

August Tarrier was the developmental editor for this book, and the best one I could possibly have had. Her decisive edits and suggestions made this a better book by encouraging me to mine more deeply the social-justice theme as it related to my personal struggles.

I am truly grateful to Julie Strauss Bettinger, fellow Goucher MFA graduate, who encouraged me to turn to Inkshares for publication of this book. Her book, *Encounters with Rikki: From Hurricane Katrina rescue to exceptional therapy dog*, is an Inkshares publication and was her thesis at Goucher. Julie is one of the most supportive writer friends an author could have.

I don't dare try to list all of the Goucher students who read and commented on my manuscript for fear of forgetting and inadvertently insulting someone. I hope a heartfelt, if general, thank you will do. But I will mention especially the members of our postdegree writers group, who have read, edited, and commented on sections of this book as well as other of my essays. Pam Kelley, Jennifer Adler, Theo Emery, Tom Kapsidelis, Jim Dahlman, Heather Bobula, Erica Johnson, and Kim Pittaway: your cogent comments and changes have made me a better writer.

And I am so very grateful for the friendships of several former Miriam's House staff members, all of whom you have met in this book. Faye Powell and I are now good friends, regularly meeting for lunch to reminisce and marvel at how far we've come. Donna Jackson is my staunch ally, a friend of the kind who seems more like family, whose sense of humor and kind attention helped me immensely after I left Miriam's House. Angie Williams is a woman of even deeper spirituality and intuition than she was fifteen years ago, a woman to admire and emulate. I possibly may have never forgiven Kathy Budzynski for leaving Miriam's House when she did—to have a baby, as though that were a good excuse—but she has forgiven me for being so difficult and is now one of my best friends, always good for easy humor and warm hospitality. Yvonne Lee and I have recently reconnected after five years apart, and, in the true test of real friendship, have picked up right where we left off with a deep and affectionate connection. David Hilfiker and I meet regularly for lunch and the best conversations to be had anywhere. I'm in a women's spirituality group with Kathy

Doan, our board president for six years, whose intelligence, passion, and sense of justice always enlighten me.

And speaking of the women's spirituality group, some of my best support comes from Rita Waters, Richelle Friedman, Gigi Gruenke, and—in past iterations of the group—Reg McCullup and Rhoda Stauffer. A special note of thanks is due to Rita, one of the first readers of the manuscript back when it was just a collection of stories. Her uncompromising assessment of certain aspects of my writing (as in, "I'm gagging here") handed me my first indication that I was allowing sentiment to overcome good craft.

Many people made a successful preorder campaign possible, earning grateful acknowledgment: N Street Village organized book events with unending enthusiasm for this memoir—Sharon Hart, Laurie Williams, Schroeder Stribling, Stuart Allen, Megan McKinley, and Gary Maring; Glenn O'Gilvie and Ericka Best at Center for Nonprofit Advancement provided wonderful preorder support; Potter's House Bookstore and Café put up a promotional poster; Amy Nelson, Abby Fenton, and Jewel Addy at Whitman Walker Health put up posters and held a book event; Kate Akalanu created the promotional video; Tommy Zarembka met with me monthly over breakfast; Nan McConnell provided early advice for my business plan; Cristina Flagg Cousins was an early reader who made helpful criticisms and then advised me on the social-media campaign; Tim Kime gave me great advice. Thanks also to individuals who worked hard for preorders: Kayla McClurg, Carolyn Arpin, David Edelfelt, Krista Sickert, Channing Wickham, Heather Marsh, Joan Marsh Sparks, and Kristen Michelle.

Thanks to Inkshares for its wonderfully democratic and writer-friendly publishing model, which I believe to be the wave of the future. Special appreciation goes to Angela Melamud and Matt Kaye, and also to Bethany Davis of Girl

Friday Productions, who did a great job coordinating editing and cover design.

And finally, I thank you, the reader, for your interest in the women of Miriam's House. My best hope is that they have, in some small way, taught you as they taught me.

ABOUT THE AUTHOR

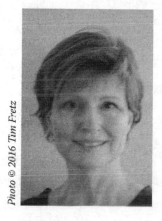

Photo © 2016 Tim Fretz

In 1996, Carol D. Marsh founded Miriam's House, a residence in Washington, DC, for homeless women living with AIDS. She lived and worked there as executive director until chronic migraine disease forced her to resign in 2009. As a way to cope with the loss of the job and community she loved, Marsh began to write stories about the women—vignettes, memorable conversations, parties, funerals, and the challenges and rewards of work that transformed her.

Marsh graduated from the master of fine arts in creative nonfiction program at Goucher College in 2014. *Nowhere Else I Want to Be* is her thesis and first book. For more information, please visit www.caroldmarsh.com and forum.caroldmarsh.com.

LIST OF PATRONS

This book was made possible in part by the following grand patrons who preordered the book on Inkshares.com. Thank you.

Amy Nelson
Ann Marie McCreedy
Ann McCreedy
Arbanet
Benjamin Sacks
Betty Good White
Byoung9071
Cagarris
Carolyn Arpin
Corriespondance
Csparks1
David Edelfelt
Dbucher53
Dorothy Larimer
Dwhilfiker
Elizabeth Stribling

Elizabeth W. Stribling
Emily Davis McCollum
Ericka Harley
Eva Pesch
Frances M. Ford
Georgia De Clark
Ginny McReynolds
Glenn O'Gilvie
Graffv5
Helen McConnell
Janel McTaggart
Joanflute
Joseph A. Budzynski
Judith D. Krueger
Julie Strauss Bettinger
Karen Brown

Karenebj

Kate Akalonu

Kathleen McCreedy

Kathy Doan

Kayla L Mcclurg

Kent R. Beduhn

Kristen

Maggyet46

Martclaa

Megan McKinley

Meridith

M.Gmaring

Mholdrich

Mikepfay

Nancy Sulfridge

Nwithbroe

Pam Kelley

Peter D. Shields

Rhoda J. Stauffer

Rose Kreider

Rosenmommy

Sallen

Shelley Marcus

Sherron L Hiemstra

Sidney W. Stolz

Stuart E Allen

Susan

Susan Galbraith

Tbrown3093

Thomas P. Kapsidelis

Timofdese

Timothy Fretz

Tracy.Cecil

Wmarsh230

Write2caro

INKSHARES

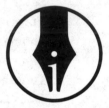

Inkshares is a crowdfunded book publisher. We democratize publishing by having readers select the books we publish—we edit, design, print, distribute, and market any book that meets a preorder threshold.

Interested in making a book idea come to life? Visit Inkshares.com to find new book projects or start your own.